Studies in Alternative Therapy 3

Communication
in and about
Alternative Therapies

Studies in
Alternative Therapy 3

Communication
in and about
Alternative Therapies

Edited by
Erling Høg and
Søren Gosvig Olesen

INRAT

Odense University Press

Studies in Alternative Therapy 3 is published in
cooperation with the International Network for
Research on Alternative Therapies (INRAT) and
sponsored by the Danish Research Council
for the Humanities (SHF).

© The Authors and Odense University Press 1996
Printed by Narayana Press, Gylling, Denmark
Cover by Ulla Poulsen Precht
ISBN 87-7838-206-8

Contents

Introduction

Søren Gosvig Olesen Erling Høg	Introduction: Communication in and about Alternative Therapies	7

Part I: Looking into the Body 9

Vilhelm Schjelderup	The Living Organism as a Biocybernetic Unity	11
Madeleine Bastide Agnès Lagache	The Paradigm of Signifiers: A Useful Tool to Analyze the Effects of Homeopathic Remedies on the Living Body	21

Part II: Medical Pluralism 35

Elisabeth Hsu	The Polyglot Practitioner: Towards Acceptance of Different Approaches in Treatment Evaluation	37
Mary Ryan-Thorup	Bridging the Domains of Sound and Symptom in Tibetan and Allopathic Medicine: Cultural Phenomenology as Praxis	54
David Aldridge	The Development of Music Therapy Research as a Perspective of Complementary Medicine	64
Helle Johannessen	Communicating Bodies – when the cell goes cultural and the doctor goes bananas	73

Part III: Homoeopathy and Placebo 83

Ursula Sharma	Building a Professional Community; Collective Culture in a Group of Non Medically Qualified Homoeopaths in Britain	85
Phillip Nicholls	A Hearing for Homoeopathy: Some Sociological Reflections on Problems of Communication about Alternative Therapy among Researchers and Practitioners	99

Toke Barfod	Four Aspects of Placebo – based on a review of the literature and a qualitative interview investigation among general practitioners and alternative therapists	111
Robert Lafaille	The Placebo: Mysterious Forces or Investigating Complexity?	127

Part IV: Researching and Networking 149

Rebecca Rees	Research and Communication: The Work of the Research Council for Complementary Medicine	151
Dieter Melchart	Integration of Complementary Medicine in Research at the University of Munich	159
Tobias Waltjen	Communication, Publication and Information Opportunities on Computer Networks – can scientific and therapeutic communities come closer together in cyberspace?	171

Part V: Dialogues and Politics 185

Motzi Eklöf	"So-called Alternative Treatment". On the medical profession's views on quackery and alternative medicine in Sweden	187
Vigdis Moe Christie	The Story of a Dialogue Group between Practitioners of Alternative (Traditional) Medicine and Modern (Western) Medicine in Norway	197
Aase K. Mortensen	Alternative Therapy and Rationality	206
Espen Braathen	Communicating the Individual Body and the Body Politic. The discourse on disease prevention and health promotion in alternative therapies	211
Bent Eikard	In the Twilight Zone. A personal report from a medical doctor betwixt and between	222

List of contributors	234

Introduction: Communication in and about Alternative Therapies

by Søren Gosvig Olesen and Erling Høg

The present volume of *Studies in Alternative Therapy* is the result of the third international INRAT seminar, held under the main heading *Communication in and about Alternative Therapies*.[1] Many different approaches are united within this theme, both those of particular disciplines and more general scientific traditions. The researchers were invited to speak on the concept of communication, not as a common general definition, but in terms of what the concept might contribute in specific areas. We would like to extend this invitation to the reader, in the hopes of continuing the dialogue started at the seminar.

The compilation of articles presented here is divided into five parts to lead the reader through different themes regarding communication research in and about health care alternatives. The purpose of this organization has been to capture different orientations within communication research, more than as a means to categorize each chapter under strictly defined themes and headings.

In Part I you will find a general, philosophical and theoretical discussion about the basis of research within the natural sciences as it is traditionally perceived. The presented ideas are articulated with special reference to changing our understanding, not merely of the natural sciences but also of the therapeutic enterprise.

Part II comprises a discussion of feasible communication between different traditions, posing the question of how we formulate the communication within the confines of a language and conceptual design, which, however, always will be 'ours'. One of the key ideas is how medical pluralism can be managed in practice, accepting different approaches in treatment evaluation, bridging realms of different medical paradigms, producing research results within complementary medicine and, not least, how to interpret and explain phenomena within different cosmologies.

---

1   The seminar "Communication in and about Alternative Therapies" took place in Værløse, Denmark, on September 29 – October 1, 1995. 34 persons from 10 different European countries and the USA were gathered, making a diverse forum of scholars from music therapy, homeopathy, immunology, medicine, anthropology, sociology, health studies, psychotherapy and philosophy. This meeting was partially sponsored by the Danish Research Council for the Humanities being a part of a four-year project, International Network for Research on Alternative Therapies (INRAT), also initiated and sponsored by the Danish Research Council for the Humanities.

Part III introduces a discussion about communication, and the lack of it, as experienced between alternative and established therapies, between researchers and practitioners, or between the therapeutic traditions and their surroundings, including the mass media. This part is primarily inspired by ideas within social theory. The case of homoeopathy in Britain emphasizes the discussion on professionalisation within a community of practitioners, followed by primarily sociological reflections on communication problems among researchers and practitioners. The complementary section of part three comprises a discussion of literature and qualitative interview research on the placebo concept in Denmark followed by a presentation of placebo within different contexts of research, history, pharmacology and complementary medicine.

Part IV sheds light on the antecedent possibilities and conditions for examining alternative treatments, seen within economic, social and information technological contexts. Research on complementary medicines has fostered different initiatives, including the emergence of research councils and networks establishing virtual communities via the electronic media. Thus, it is very important to present a few concrete examples of how such initiatives contribute communicative means to health care research. This section thus includes information about a London based research council on complementary medicine, a specific research initiative in Germany emphasizing the need for more research and databases to ease the relationship between different research communities and medical insurance companies, and also some reflections on how scientific and therapeutic communities might take advantage of available electronic media.

The cultural context for the research based articles presented in the fifth and final part of this book is clearly Scandinavian, as the authors come from Sweden, Norway and Denmark. This part examines the political forum for communication in and about health care alternatives, both as this forum appears from more official arenas, and as it has been experienced through activities and co-operation at a grass roots level. This political question applies to researchers, politicians and lobbyists, but is also meant as a diplomatic means for enriching the public tone and communiqué with and about alternative treatment.

Taken together, the presented articles shed light on the difficult conditions for communication in and about alternative therapies. In any case, it is probably an essential part of its nature that any communication is inclusive as well as excluding. In other words, meaning can only be presented and given a more explicit formulation when different meaning is eliminated. Does this also imply, as many a chapter within the history and research on alternative therapies possibly suggests, that in-communication is a more basic dimension than mere communication?

Part I

Looking into the Body

The Living Organism as a Biocybernetic Unity

by Vilhelm Schjelderup

A number of complementary therapies are based on the common principle that the whole organism is found projected in a circumscribed part of the body. These therapies have been classified as either acupuncture microsystems, or as somatotopic, holographic, or bioholographic methods. They have proved useful in clinical practice, being used in the treatment of millions of patients yearly, and they are now gaining world-wide recognition.

Apparently these methods reflect a general physiological principle: a kind of holographic mirroring of the whole organism in its parts. It is a dynamic, two-way relationship: A pathological change in the whole organism is reflected in corresponding changes in each of the microsystems, and a therapeutic intervention in one of the microsystems may affect a corresponding change in the whole organism. That is why we can use these methods both for diagnostic and therapeutic purposes.

The common nature of these methods suggests that they are due to a general biological principle. Until recently, however, we have had no general biological science allowing us to explore the full implications of this holographic structuring of living beings. Such a new theory has now been developed in China and is presented as a new discipline of biology and medicine under the name of ECIWO biology.

ECIWO Biology

ECIWO biology has been founded by Professor Yinqing Zhang of Shandong University in China. It is based on the hypothesis that a living organism actually constitutes a multilevel mosaic, where each unit contains the information of the whole organism, and has an embryonic potential which we call totipotental. In the term "ECIWO" the "E" stands for embryo, the "C" for containing, the "I" for information, the "W" for whole, and the "O" for organism. The idea is that each part of the organism, representing a certain degree of unity, contains the information of the whole organism, and has the potential of turning into a fetus that may generate a new organism of the same kind (Zhang 1990).

For plants this embryonic totipotential of the part is well documented from empirical facts. If we take a branch of a tree, or even a twig or a leaf, and plant it into the soil, it may develop roots and grow into a new tree of the same kind. Each of these parts, the branch, the twig and the leaf, represent an embryonic unity – or as we say in ECIWO biology "an ECIWO" – at a different organic level. That is why we say that a living organism constitutes a multilevel mosaic of ECIWOs. The lowest level is the cell and the highest level is the whole organism. The cell and the whole organism accordingly represent special cases of an ECIWO in ECIWO biology.

In the case of lower animals it is also well known that a part may turn into a fetus generating a new individual. If we cut an earthworm into appropriate pieces, for example, each part may grow into a new earthworm. In higher animals the embryonic potential of the part to generate a new individual has been lost or is suppressed. According to ECIWO theory, the part, however, still contains the information of the whole organism, and it has an embryonic potential which is found expressed in a regenerative potential acting on the whole organism.

This regenerative aspect of ECIWO totipotency is of great significance to medicine, both in its practical applications and in its theoretical implications. It gives us a new understanding of the biological relation between the whole organism and its parts, and it provides us with a new scientific basis to explain regenerative and healing processes.

During the 1980s four congresses of ECIWO biology were held in China. The first international congress was held in Singapore in 1990 and the second in Oslo in 1992. In his address to the congress in Singapore Hu Ximing, Vice-Minister of Public Health of China and Director of State Administration of Traditional Chinese Medicine, stated:

> "The founding of the ECIWO theory and ECIWO biology is one of the most important events in the history of biology in this century. It will bring about a conceptual change in our understanding of the organism. It will exert an important influence upon the development of biology and medicine, especially upon the modernization of traditional medicine such as Traditional Chinese Medicine. . . . Today ECIWO biology is widely applied to medicine, zoology, botany, Chinese herbal medicine, horticulture, paleontology, cancer study and some other realms" (Hu 1990: 1).

Very few studies have been completed comparing the therapeutic efficacy of different schools of medicine. One of these few was carried out by Huang Jiqun, chief physician of Xinfeng Hospital of Traditional Chinese Medicine in Jianxi, China. It comprised 3,400 patients in a parallel study, comparing the results obtained in the treatment of common medical problems, like infantile diarrhea, acute hepatitis, common cold, dysmenorrhea, fracture pain and pain due to soft tissue injury, for patients treated with either Western medicine, traditional Chinese medicine or ECIWO medicine. In this study ECIWO medicine came out best for all groups of medical disorders, except for acute hepatitis where equally good results were obtained with ECIWO medicine and traditional Chinese medicine, the group treated with Western medicine trailing far behind (Zhang 1991: 45-46). Such studies should be repeated in other countries and under other medical and scientific conditions. This study from China may, however, be taken as an indication that ECIWO methods compete well in ordinary clinical medicine.

In this paper I will discuss how the bioholographic methods that have been developed in practical medicine confirm the ECIWO hypothesis; how biocybernetic concepts may contribute to a better understanding of ECIWO biology; and how ECIWO biology may give us a new understanding of organic unity. In this last discussion I will try to show how the basic postulates of ECIWO biology actually exemplify the fundamental metaphysical dialectics of Plato as we find it in his dialogue "Parmenides".

Bioholographic Methods

ECIWO theory explains the different bioholographic methods that have been discovered in practical medicine, as pertaining to different ECIWOs of the body. These methods, like ear acupuncture and foot reflexology, are based on the common principle that the various organs and parts of the organism are reflected cartographically as points or small zones within the boundaries of a circumscribed part of the body. These zones are found to be in a significant physiological relationship to the corresponding organs, a relationship which is utilized for diagnostic and therapeutic purposes.

Writing about these bioholographic methods in 1982, I wrote:

> "It is striking to see how these different methods founded on the same principle have been developed in different parts of the world on empirical grounds. Although the validity of some of them may be disputed, the collective evidence indicates that such a holographic principle must be of great and largely unexplored medical importance and have a biological significance that merits further discussion" (Schjelderup 1982: 168-169).

Since 1982 more such bioholographic methods have become known, and quite a lot more clinical and experimental evidence has been gathered. Such methods have been discovered for the external ear (ear acupuncture and ear medicine); the nose and the nasal mucosa (nose acupuncture and nasal reflex therapy); the hands (hand acupuncture and hand reflexology); the feet (foot reflexology); the scalp (old and new scalp acupuncture); the retroauricular and the jugular areas (Yamamoto's new scalp acupuncture); the teeth and dental mucosa (the oral acupuncture of Jochen Gleditsch); the retromolar area (Jochen Gleditsch); the iris (iridology); and the periorbital area (eye acupuncture).

These methods, that have been discovered and developed independently of ECIWO biology, have proven highly effective in clinical medicine. ECIWO biology has added new similar methods, like Yingqing Zhang's second metacarpal system, and given these bioholographic methods a broader scientific basis in biological theory (Zhang 1990 and 1991). All these methods are in accordance with the ECIWO principles, exemplifying how the part contains the information of the whole organism, how corresponding zones of the different ECIWOs are related by the bioholographic law, and how the part has embryonic properties and may exert a regenerative effect on the whole. Taken together, these methods offer a very strong scientific argument for the ECIWO hypothesis and provide a huge amount of clinical and experimental evidence for its medical significance.

Biocybernetic Function

In bioholographic diagnosis there are two main parameters we use to identify an affected zone in an ECIWO, corresponding to an ailing part of the whole organism. The first of these is increased pain sensitivity to pressure. The other is increased electroactivity, in general a marked decrease in electrical skin resistance.

From a biocybernetic point of view the increased sensitivity of affected bioholographic zones to pressure may serve a biological purpose. If we, for example, look at the zones of foot reflexology, these zones will continuously be massaged when we walk. Operationally, this means that the increased sensitivity of affected zones may selectively serve to strengthen the corresponding ailing parts of the body by a feed back mechanism. A similar biocybernetic function will apply also to other ECIWOs, or bioholographic systems, of the body. The bioholographic zone systems apparently have an important biological function, serving to restore homeostasis and stimulate regenerative processes where these are needed in the living organism.

The increased electrical conductivity of affected bioholographic points may serve a similar purpose. Looking at it from a bioelectrical point of view, the body may be sucking up wanted electrons from the surroundings, or discharging superfluous electrons, through these points. The increased electroactivity of affected bioholographic points may in this way serve a biocybernetic function promoting homeostasis and regenerative processes in the living body. A prerequisite for such a hypothesis would be that we have a bioelectrical system in the body regulating homeostasis and regenerative processes, and that this system accounts for the electroactivity of bioholographic zones.

Such a bioelectrical system has in fact been discovered by the American orthopedic surgeon, Robert Becker. Measuring electrical skin potentials during the regeneration of amputated forelegs in salamanders, Becker discovered in 1958 a negative electrical current concurrent with the regenerative phase. Through his further research Becker discovered that this "regenerative" current is a direct electrical current of semiconductive type that is mediated by the nervous system. It is, however, not mediated by the nerves and nervous cells proper, but by the Schwann cells of the peripherous nervous system and the glial and ependymal cells of the central nervous system (Becker 1985). It is thus a perineural system, and it apparently serves as an analog electrical information system, regulating regenerative and healing processes in the body.

This bioelectrical system, based on semiconductor electricity which Becker has discovered, may well explain the electroactivity of bioholographic points. We therefore have reason to conclude that both the increased sensitivity to pressure and the increased electroactivity of affected bioholographic points serve biocybernetic functions. Such a biocybernetic function may not be restricted to the physical modalities of pressure and electricity. Other physical stimuli may play a similar role, exerting a biocybernetic effect on the organism through the bioholographic zone systems.

From a biological point of view these biocybernetic functions of the bioholographic organization of the organism must be of very great significance. They help to explain the great resilience of living organisms, and how living systems in spite of far greater complexity may outlast mechanical ones. This built-in, biocybernetic resilience of living organisms explains how we actually preserve and strengthen our health through activity and interaction with our surroundings. ECIWO theory supports a dynamic view of human health.

A Biophysical Explanation?

The biocybernetic properties of living organisms, due to their structuring according to ECIWO principles, explain their functional strength and adaptability and must be of great biological significance. We see how a living organism functionally is knit into a dynamic wholeness where the whole organism and its different parts intimately respond to each other and reinforce each other to create what we might call a tightly bound organic unity.

If this may be a part of the answer to the biological question of "how?" posed by ECIWO biology, it is, however, not an exhaustive answer to the even more significant scientific question of "why?". What is the deeper meaning of ECIWO biology? Why do we discover that living organisms are composed in this way of parts that contain both the information and the potential of the whole?

In 1982 discussing the biological significance of the bioholograhic principle, I tried to answer this question on the basis of physical holography and the physics of wave functions:

> "In mathematics the theory of holography belongs to the classical theory of partial coherence. In the physics of radiation a hologram is created as an interference pattern between the difracted radiation from an object and a coherent background, like a standing wave. From a part of this hologram the image of the original object may be reconstructed by physical or mathematical means. Actually, any part of the hologram contains the information of the whole object, only the sharpness of the reconstructed image will depend on the size of the part.
>
> In the holographic methods we encounter in medicine, the organism as a whole is seen projected as a kind of hologram on a part of the organism, as the external ear, the nasal mucosa, the feet, the hands, the scalp, the irises or the large intestine. This holographic pattern again reflects back on the organism as a whole. It is this two-way holographic process – or this dynamic holography, as we may call it – which constitutes the basis for the use of these methods both for diagnostic and for therapeutic purposes.
>
> The holographic process is thus seen to serve a double function: to impress the message of the whole on the part, and then by a feedback mechanism to let the whole respond to a change in the part. Such a double function will obviously serve the purpose of biological organization: how the organism, which to the analytical eye is seen to be composed of an infinite number of parts, may as yet function as a whole and preserve internal coherence. This great, unsolved problem of biological organization and coherence will pose enormous demands to any physical explanation and would require the utmost from any mathematical theory of partial coherence. We should indeed not be surprised to find that this startling child of mathematical physics, the science of holography, may have an important part to play in this connection.

The ability to utilize holographic processes may thus be a fundamental property of living organisms. We should expect it to be an intrinsic mechanism in embryological development, a means by which the embryological plan of the organism is worked out. Dr. Nogier's image of the human ear and the embryo would thus convey a double insight: that of the projection of the organism in the ear, and that of the fundamental significance of the holographic principle in the embryological development.

In physics the principle of holography is a consequence of the wave properties of physical reality. If the holographic systems that have been discovered in medical practice, really represent holographic patterns in a physical sense, they must be explained on the basis of a biophysical theory which accounts for biological wave patterns. Such biophysical theories have recently been developed" (Schjelderup 1982: 169).

A main argument against an explanation of the bioholographic systems based on physical holography and a biophysical theory of biological wave patterns, is that the bioholographic patterns do not conform to what we usually perceive as physical holograms. This argument is, however, not decisive. Physical holography may still account for how such bioholographic patterns were developed early in embryological development, or indeed during the early development of life on this planet. In the theory of bioplasma, as it has been developed by Professor V. Injushin, holographic processes are an integrated part of the biophysical structure of living organisms. And at an even deeper physical level the ECIWO structuring of living organisms may be explained on the basis of David Bohm's theory of the implicate order and holomovements (Bohm 1980). Bohm's theory may even provide us with a physical explanation of the medical effects of high potency homeopathy, as I have tried to show (Schjelderup 1989). It is thus possible on the basis of the theory of implicate order to develop a scientific theory of healing processes that embraces both the bioholographic methods of ECIWO biology and homeopathy.

Wholeness and Unity

An investigation into the possible physical basis of ECIWO biology in holography and the wave properties of physical reality certainly is relevant. I have, however, come to the conclusion that such a biophysical explanation will not be sufficient to explain the "why?" of the ECIWO principles. It may to a large extent explain the wholeness of living organisms, and how the part relates to the whole and the whole to its parts. But it will not give a sufficient explanation of the unity of a living organism.

A living organism constitutes a whole. But even more basic to our understanding of a living being is its unity. It is this unity of a living organism which is the basis for its uniqueness, and the fact that we may regard it as a subject in its confrontation with an external world. Wholeness implies the concept of unity. But wholeness is something that is composite of parts, and unity by definition is something singular. Implicit in our understanding of what a living organism is, we are thus faced with a logical paradox which needs clarification.

A solution of this paradox is beyond what has generally been considered biological science. This problem actually belongs to philosophy and metaphysics. It may, however, be deeply relevant to our understanding of ECIWO biology and its more profound scientific implications.

The classical exposition of this paradox is found in Plato's dialogue "Parmenides". In this dialogue Plato explores the logical relations between the two basic metaphysical ideas of "unity" and "being". Let us explore the logical consequences of the second hypothesis of "Parmenides": *"If the one is"* – that is, if unity has being or existence – it follows that *"number is"* and *"the straight and the broken line"* (Plato: "Parmenides" 142B1-153E3): meaning that reality has a mathematical structure. The second and the fourth hypotheses of "Parmenides" (*"if the one is, what must then necessarily be the consequences for the other(s)-than-the-one"*) (Plato: "Parmenides" 157B6-159B1) thus give the metaphysical foundation for the rational and mathematical structure of physical reality which has been explored in science.

For our discussion it is important that Plato in his logical analysis of the consequences of the second and fourth hypotheses of "Parmenides" actually removes the basis for the wholeness/part axiom of Euclid's geometry. This axiom states that no part can be equal to the whole of which it is a part. Just as the strict mathematical necessity of the parallel axiom of Euclid was disproved by Riemann in 1840, the wholeness/part axiom was finally disproved by the German mathematician Cantor by the end of last century. Riemann's geometry forms the basis for the geometrical formulation of Einstein's general theory of relativity, and Cantor's group theory has become an equally essential mathematic tool for 20th century physics. Hermann Weyl's classic *The Theory of Groups and Quantum Mechanics* is probably still the most elegant mathematical formulation of quantum theory in existence.

A part is not, as Plato shows in the fourth hypothesis of "Parmenides", just a part of "all" parts, but a part of a whole. If there is no wholeness, there are no parts, just a sum of separate things. The concept of "wholeness" may imply different meanings. But if we look at a living organism, it constitutes a unity that cannot be explained by the combination of its parts. Rather, as we see from ECIWO biology, the whole organism and the different ECIWOs of which it is composed, belong to the same group of group theory. The whole organism is just a special case of an ECIWO, as we learn in ECIWO biology. And each part, or ECIWO, contains the information, i.e., the pattern, of the whole.

This relationship between the whole and its parts is what we call "holomeric" (from *holon* meaning whole, and *meros* meaning part). In this holomeric relation the part is not only a part of the whole, but the whole is also a part of each of its parts, giving the part a structure or pattern of the whole (Wyller 1981). This is exactly the relation we find in ECIWO biology between the whole organism and its parts. For this reason it would be scientifically more accurate to use the term "holomeric" instead of "holographic" to designate this relationship in ECIWO biology.

Plato gives a metaphysical foundation for this holomeric relation in his exposition of the second hypothesis of "Parmenides". If unity, which strictly speaking is "beyond" being, takes part in being, it will establish together with being a plurality consisting of two elements, "unity" and "being". And being a composite, this can be divided into parts, each part necessarily having both "unity" and "being". Each part will thus constitute a new unity, having the same pattern of wholeness, and at the same time be a composite that can be further divided. According to the fourth hypothesis of "Parmenides", this will be the structure of physical beings as a consequence of their partaking of the "one", i.e., of their having unity.

In "Parmenides" Plato thus gives us a metaphysical framework for solving the biological paradox of a living organism at the same time being a unity and a composite of parts. We see that such a solution would be in agreement with ECIWO biology. The findings of ECIWO biology may thus inspire new thought on the fundamental scientific and philosophical basis of biology. Incidentally, Plato in "Parmenides" also answers the Aristotelian criticism of his theory of ideas, at the same time laying the metaphysical foundation for a better theory. ECIWO biology thus touches on profound questions implicit in the tradition of Western philosophy. It may thus not only inspire a renewal of Chinese medical and philosophical thought, but also a renewal in Western biology and philosophy. Here possibly East and West may meet in a new understanding of life and its relation to the universe.

References

Becker, Robert O.
1985   *The Body Electric*, William Morrow and Co.: New York.

Bohm, David
1980   *Wholeness and the Implicate Order*, Routledge and Kegan Paul: London.

Hu, Ximing
1990   "Congress address" in: *Progress in ECIWO Biology*, pp. 1-2, Higher Education Press: Beijing.

Plato
380 B.C.? "Parmenides".

Schjelderup, Vilhelm
1982   "The principle of holography: a key to a holistic approach in medicine", in: *American Journal of Acupuncture*, 10(2): 167-171.
1989   *Nytt lys på medisinen*, pp. 252-260, J.W. Cappelen: Oslo.

Wyller, Egil A.
1981   *Enhet og annethet*, pp. 222-231, Dreyers Forlag: Oslo.

Zhang, Yingqing
1990   "An outline of the ECIWO theory" in: *Progress in ECIWO Biology*, pp. 51-264, Higher Education Press: Beijing.
1991   *ECIWO and its Application to Medicine*, Shandong Science and Technology Press: China.

The Paradigm of Signifiers: A Useful Tool to Analyze the Effects of Homeopathic Remedies on the Living Body

by Madeleine Bastide and Agnès Lagache

The mechanistic paradigm has been so fruitful that we think it is the only law of rationality. However, other facts necessitate the creation of new ways of thinking, though we still need to be rational. Each kind of interaction has its own logical modalities. Just as the mechanistic paradigm seizes the material interactions between objects and the symbolic paradigm assumes linguistic facts, we need a paradigm that allows for the understanding of living structures. As such, we can present the paradigm of signifiers (Lagache 1988; Bastide & Lagache 1992; Bastide et al 1995: 237; Bastide & Lagache 1996): *"Living beings communicate with their world in a nonverbal way, whether on a somatic or psychological level."* This paradigm takes place within the framework of the logic of analogy. It introduces the real effect of "semantic objects" and the general law of its transmission. Its application can be used to interpret homeopathic experimentation or the therapeutic effects of homeopathy. It is also very useful in understanding immunological concepts.

The Living Body as an Informed-Informing Structure

Our way of thinking is inherited from positivism: *"Everything is matter, according to the very restricted definition of the matter provided by the mechanistic paradigm. Consequently, it was thought that every problem (or every object) was solvable by reducing its terms (or itself) into simple material elements. Matter rules over everything"* (Lagache 1996a). The mechanistic materialism transformed the positive method into philosophical and social totalitarian practice. If we consider the properties of the object according to the mechanistic paradigm, it is homogenous and it may be separated into its different elements; it does not change except by wear of time; it changes only in terms of its spatial position and it is characterized by autarchy. The object responds to thermodynamic laws and is, by approximation, not related to its environment; it is a physicochemical material (Bastide & Lagache 1992). These characteristics are not acceptable for the living body.

On the contrary, the living body is heterogenous and cannot be separated into its different elements as it functions as a whole. This represents a major difficulty for biological science. Interrelationships between the different biological systems of the body are so strong that the body must be considered as a whole. However, scientists traditionally have always been disturbed by the problem of individual biological systems. Moreover, the living body is different before and after the events that it comes across and it is continuously modified as a function of time. The body has a psychological memory as well as a physical one, as shown by the immune system: it learns how to fight against aggressions and remember them. Even bacteria and isolated cells are able to organize their defence after the recognition of an aggression as it may be observed in the hormetic model. The living bodies are in a continual and irreversible learning process. They show interactions at every level from psychic to physical as demonstrated for example in psycho-neuro-immunology. They are never independent from their environment and are in continuous relationship with the external world (see figure 1). Therefore, the body is able to receive *information*. The living body is neither an object nor an idea and needs to communicate with the environment (Lagache 1996b).

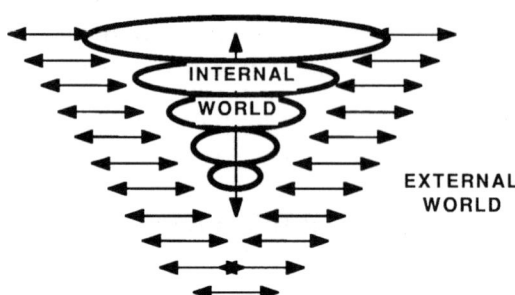

Figure 1: The living body, an informed-informing structure

The living body (body and mind) is a complex structure with different levels of information. It is able to exchange information with the external world. Information also circulates in the internal world allowing exchanges at every level. The living body has the ability to deal with information at the right level.

We now have to give a definition of *information*. According to Bateson's definition, information is *"a difference which makes a difference"* (Bateson 1977). A piece of information is not an object, whatever the medium used to transfer it. *"A lost jigsaw piece in a children's room has no meaning, except to make the difference between a tidy and untidy home. Putting it in its jigsaw's frame with the other pieces makes a new meaning arise: It was this pretty star which was lacking in the sky in the left corner . . . Sense is an emigrant, the new and impalpable dimension which arises not from objects, but from the network of relationships woven around objects"* (Lagache 1996b). Information is an event able to modify a receiver in an irreversible way (even in a short term). It is the receiver that creates the event as a significant element modifying its own behaviour. The result of information is only observed in the receiver and depends on the capacity of the receiver to read and treat this information: the receiver is usually active. Information is only read in a context which makes sense of the information and therefore becomes significant to the receiver. Meaning is nonlocal: it assumes movement in a large and multiple network including different environments. No meaning is described in a closed or isolated system. These pieces of information which have meaning are designated as signifiers. Sense has its source in simple facts: affect of the self, modification by an element that produces an event for the whole; expansion of the environment in which the affect of the self may make sense for another receiver. One can take as an example animal mimetism: the affect of the self is first a passive mimesis, the external environment invades the interior world and determines it; nevertheless, a wide focusing is enough to introduce the predator, in order for the mimesis to become active: the affect of the self becomes a signal, or in this case a "non-signal" signifier, a dissimulation in the predator's eyes.

This communication is essentially a *mediation* between a living being and its world, and also a mediation between one state of the living being and another. The notion of *mediation is a general concept* which links two states, or two phenomena, in a dynamic way, creating a new level (acquisition, or transformation, or evolution etc.). It may concern two different things whose relationship has traditionally been ignored. In modern science, body and mind are two separate things, each one isolated in its own camp. Attempts to join them together exist, but the symbolic paradigm is unable to explain objects (function of molecules, biochemistry of physiological regulations, etc.). The mechanistic paradigm would like to explain mind, memory and behavior and consciousness exclusively in terms of interactions between molecules and receptors. A good example is given by psycho-neuro-immunology where one part of the research analyses the interactions of neuropeptides with the immune system and another part studies immunological products like cytokines and their interactions with the nervous system or on behavior. It is quite difficult to approach the real synthesis between these events.

On the contrary, mediation creates a link which differentiates each element. *"We need something which links mind and body, creating a bridge between physical and semantic facts, whilst maintaining the distance and difference between them: that is a mediation"* (Lagache 1996a). Mediation takes place before the objects that arise from it: it is a creative element which enables different levels of reality to exist according to their own identity, while working together in nature. This concept of mediation provides a way to understand creative organizations and temporal regulations (Lagache 1996). It may be applied to any separated elements which may be related by this constructive concept creating a bridge. The paradigm of signifiers is itself a mediation between the mechanistic paradigm and the symbolic one (see figure 2). The logic of information exchange does not follow the same rules as an exchange of objects where one loses and the other gains; the exchange of information creates a new situation which is not the sum of exchanges. *"It is a dynamic process, through which the partners change and build themselves by dealing with information: the very mediation creates what it mediates. Reasoning in terms of mechanistic elements is not enough to understand life, but we assume that: first, living structures imply mechanical organization combined with semantic facts; second, mediations are the dynamic elements which make living structures work as a whole"* (Lagache 1996b). We can therefore consider semantic objects as pieces of information which call for a processing and active regulation by the whole system.

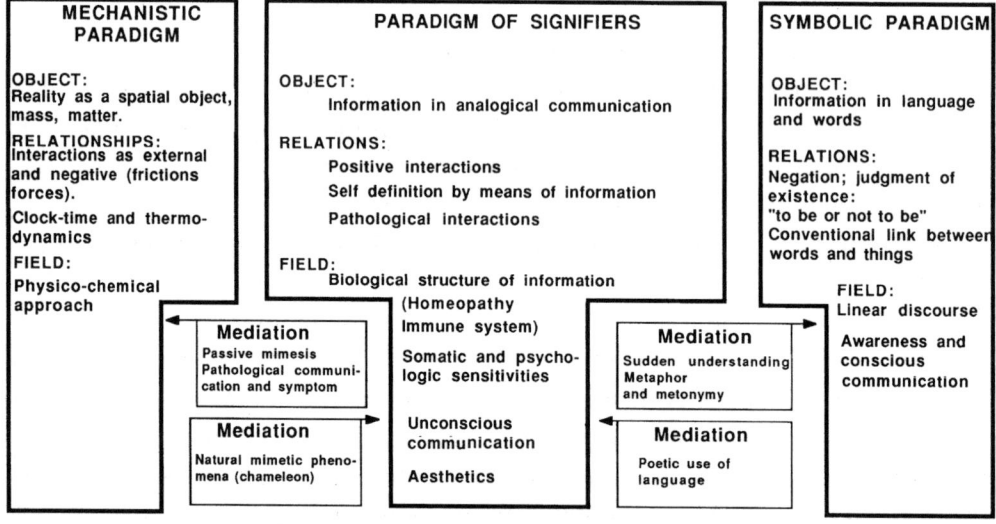

Figure 2: Epistemological classification of paradigms

We will see below that the pathological symptom is a mediation which allows the physician to understand the meaningful unity of the disease. In the same way, the diluted homeopathic remedy creating the description of the pathogenetic symptom in a healthy subject is also a mediation which will be able to reinform the patient showing the same symptoms. Examples of mediations are given by psychoanalysis and Freudian concepts which reveal the somatization of psychological facts.

The Semantic Object

The *semantic object is a concrete element, neither symbolic nor linguistic but treated by the body as a piece of information*. It fulfills the function of a mediation. The semantic object (or physical signifier) may induce a learning process which may be memorized by the living organism. It will transfer information to the living body. The body will then deal with this information and modify its behavior accordingly.

The circulation of this type of *semantic object* has its own original laws (of which we sketched the description, Lagache 1988). It looks like an analogical communication, as we find them for example in aesthetics, psychoanalysis, and in some features of modern logic and linguistics. Here we will simply point out three eminent characteristics:

1) The piece of information is not an object even if it has a *carrier*. It is an event (first difference), able to modify a receiver in an irreversible way (even for a short term); it is the receiver that creates the event, as a significant element modifying its own circumstances (second difference). Thus, information is *"a difference which makes a difference"* (Bateson 1977).

2) Meaning is nonlocal: it assumes movement in a large and multiple network including different environments. No meaning is describable for a closed or isolated system.

3) The simplest mode of representation for living structures is a passive mimesis: one external modification is reproduced as an affect of the self. For example, the median line on the fish represents its water motions. However, this representation is an internal event. It interacts there with a new set, able then to deal with information, to react with its own idiosyncrasy.

The semantic object materially designates information to be transmitted as a signifier for the body to deal with.

Function of the Semantic Objects

An example is given by aesthetics in which concrete phenomena (music, painting) are meaningful to the body. Aldridge provides an extreme example by using music in therapy applied to coma patients and victims of Alzheimer's disease (Aldridge 1989, 1990, 1993). In this approach, the body receives musical information within a rhythmic context of communication which enables healing to take place. In the above cases, the musical components are fundamental to the body's communication and these play a role by their rhythmicity. According to the level of pathology, different levels of rhythmicity as carriers of information may act upon the body and represent different levels of semantic objects.

In order to communicate, the living organism needs to establish a representation of the world. The simplest way for it to do this is by using an analogical model designated by mimesis. This means that the image of the object is the easiest representation and the only possible one. We can then describe the most fascinating operation of the living receiver as the general form of the *active mimesis*. The living organism is capable of receiving the semantic object, not as a material object but as information about this object. It already calls for a processing and active regulation by the whole system.

We consider, for example, that a diluted succussed solution prepared with a chemical carries the mimetic representation of the effects of that chemical on the healthy body. This effect on the healthy body is described as pathogenetic symptoms used in *similia principle* in homeopathy. When the organism receives the information that corresponds to its symptomatic manifestation, it recognizes it and deals with it. Consequently, regulatory effects will occur by modifying the symptoms of the body, if the representation brought by the succussed remedy is relevant to the symptoms, i.e., if the similarity is good. According to the *similia principle*, the homeopathic remedy is the mimetic representation of disease. Some conditions must be fulfilled. The object has to be alleviated, artificial, diluted, "light" enough not to pour in a material determination. If it is in a significant relationship with the receiver's referents, this one receives the semantic object on a higher level of organization, as treatable information, understandable, made negative if need be. This information is carried by succussed homeopathic dilutions: The information of the remedy is not related to the presence of the molecules but to the passage of information given by the molecules after dilution and succussion.

This curative effect is designated as *active mimesis*, which means that the organism was able to treat the information and to modify itself by switching to *new normal state*. This process is designated by paradoxical negation, which means that the symptoms disappear once the body receives and deals with information.

The method used to reach this point is related to the level of information.

When the organism is able to receive and recognize the information but is not able to treat it, we observe a *passive mimesis* which looks as if the symptoms have increased rather than been corrected (worsening effect). Examples of worsening are currently observed in experimental models based on the activity of endogenous molecules.

These points have raised the question of the regulatory effect of active mimesis which is organized according to the level of information. This hierarchy is organized according to the level of complexity of information.

Examples of Succussed High Dilutions as Semantic Objects

We will validate the use of the paradigm of signifiers by demonstrating the effects of semantic objects in experimental models.

Hormesis and the law of identity
The most simple learning process is the hormetic model. This phenomenon implies an opposite effect of high concentrations (toxic effect) and low concentrations (stimulating effect) (figure 3a). It is the most classical model allowing to demonstrate the biological effect of high dilutions (Bastide 1996a). As an example, a pharmacological compound like aspirin will induce a specific effect when received in allopathic concentration. This effect is received as an aggression by the body. High dilutions of aspirin have induced the opposite effect allowing the defence of the organism against the aggression of ponderal concentrations of the remedy. Effectively, it has been observed (Doutremepuich *et al* 1994) that high dilutions of aspirin had a statistically significant thrombogenic effect which corresponds to the opposite classical therapeutic effect which is anti-thombogenic when used in ponderal concentrations.

Pretreatment by low concentrations of poison have been used in cell models in various living organisms to decrease the poisoning effect. This is designated traditionally by "mithridatization". Heavy metals have been used, or arsenite, or many other products. This situation is typically a learning process with or without a short memory (figure 3b). The living organism (from procaryots to insects and to mammals) prepares its defence according to the nature of the aggression: A heavy metal needs heat shock proteins as a specific defence effect and increases the vitality of the organisms or the cells. Weis & Weis (1986) showed that, after cadmium intoxication of fish, fin regeneration occurred more rapidly if a pretreatment with a lower dose of cadmium had been applied. Van Wijk *et al* (1993, 1994) tried to analyse the general cellular adaptation syndrome by using cellular models. All the events described concern the adaptive process during the cell cycle after toxic (arsenite) treatment related to the action of heat shock proteins. The general observation of a stimulation of life and longevity has been observed after hormetic stimulation by toxic substances (Oberbaum & Cambar 1994).

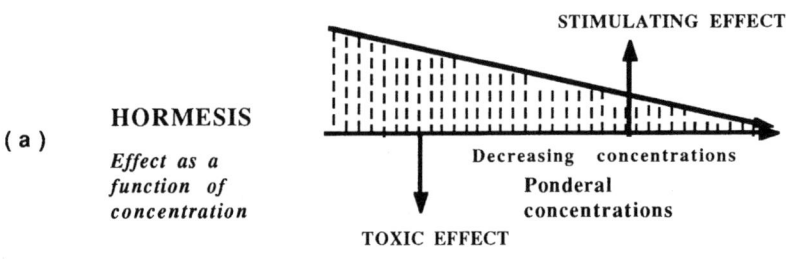

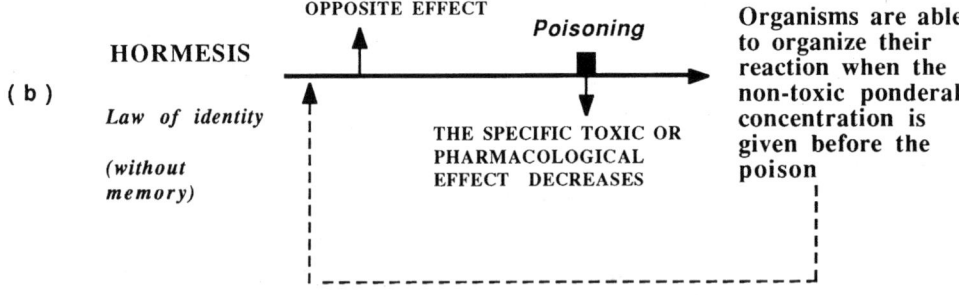

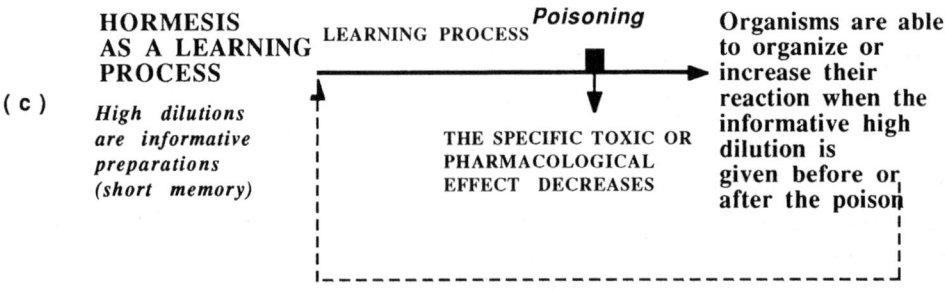

Figure 3: Interpretation of the hormetic model

The same observations have been made by researchers using succussed high dilutions of the poison itself (figure 3c). This may be observed either with pretreatment or after poisoning: In the first case, the living organism is, as before, in a learning process; in the second case, the defence is increased by an addition of information. Succussed high dilutions are supposed to be an informing structure. Examples of protection by succussed high dilutions of heavy metal are given by using 10^{-30} or 10^{-40}M of cadmium or cis-platinum (Delbancut 1994).

We propose that pretreatment by high dilutions allows a true learning process aimed at establishing a protection against the "waited danger". Specific appropriate tools are conceived and performed by the living organism in order to fight against the aggression. When the low dose is given after the toxic challenge, it allows an amplification of the organized defence, helping its achievement.

Effect of high dilutions of endogenous molecules
Some experimental models are performed by using high dilutions of endogenous molecules, belonging to the organism itself. The information is automatically read thanks to genomic structure. It is easy now to understand that a framework for understanding is necessary in order to observe an "effect" of this information. Many experimental models have been carried out with endogenous molecules, most of them relevant to the immune system. Descriptions of an immunomodulatory activity of succussed dilutions of bursin or thymulin are described (Bastide & Boudard 1996, Youbicier-Simo *et al* 1993). We have tested molecules isolated from the immune system: thymic hormones which induce intra- or extra-thymic maturation of the T lymphocytes in humans or mammals, bursin which participates in B lymphocyte maturation in the bursa of Fabricius of aves [2] and cytokines which take part in cellular interactions. Although most of our investigations were carried out with thymulin and natural mouse leucocytary interferon which it contained, we sometimes tested other thymic hormones (thymosin and thymopoïetin), and interleukin 2 (IL-2). Investigating the activity of such different kinds of molecules, we were able to verify the specificity of the information they transmitted. Highly diluted histamine or the highly diluted antigen itself was also administered in isolated hearts of guinea pigs immunized with ovalbumin: they induced significant coronary flow variations (Hadji 1992). Thyroxine was administered in highly diluted succussed solution (10^{-30}) to frogs at the end of the metamorphosis. Significant modifications of the motility were observed (Endler *et al* 1994). In these models, high dilutions bring information of endogenous molecules which are automatically recognized by the living organism (whole body or organ). The effects of this endogenous molecule information belong to various mechanisms according to the nature and the level of information and the state of the receiver.

These results are significant. In these three models, the information was clearly read by the receiver and the living structure was able to treat this information. The possibility of a strong worsening effect exists if there is a misunderstanding which will cause a passive mimesis. The clearer the information, the better the correcting effect. An organism that is too weak or a piece of information that is too powerful can provoke irreversible worsening effects.

Homeopathy and the similia principle
The diluted succussed remedy chosen according to the pathogenesy of the remedy (which describes the symptoms observed after administration of this remedy to a healthy patient) is prescribed according to the *similia principle* (figure 4). The more similar the symptoms of the patient and the remedy are, the more effective the remedy. The medical device has to reinform the patient and make his symptoms move on towards a higher level of integration. The dilution of the remedy permits us to read it as information about disease. Symptoms can be recognized as an erroneous adaptation of the organism, engaged in a process of paradoxical negation. The action of the remedies consists of a dynamic analogy between pieces of information (Lagache 1988, Bastide & Lagache 1992, Bastide *et al* 1995).

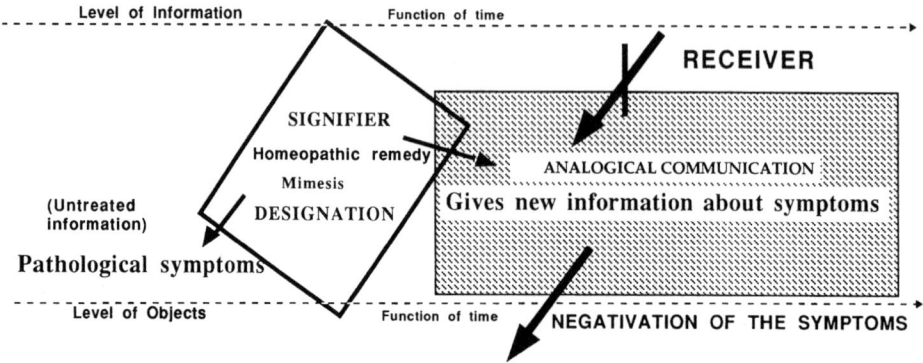

Figure 4: Therapeutic effect by application of the similia law

Conclusion

The application of the paradigm of signifiers to the homeopathic model is determined by the relationship between several parameters due to the informative ability of the remedy and the level of organization of the receiver (figure 5).

The power of the homeopathic remedy is related to its capacity to be recognized as a signifier by the receiver in a mimetic function; an exogenous remedy needs to be evaluated by a pathogenesy (effect of ponderal doses on a healthy subject) in order to establish the mimetic function of the remedy. However, an endogenous remedy (which belongs to the self molecules) will be automatically recognized by the receiver.

The dilutions which contain the successively diluted succussed solutions of molecules increase the informative ability by transforming the "object-remedy" into an informing preparation which can be understood by the receiver as a signifier.

The organization of the receiver is linked to its capacity to perceive the information of the remedy: the higher the mimetic function, the stronger the effect as in the "sensitive types"; regarding endogenous molecules, the higher their function in the hierarchy of the living system, the stronger the effect. The effect of the information given by endogenous molecules can be misunderstood when the information is not targeted, and a worsening effect may occur.

The regulating effect of the homeopathic remedy prescribed according to the similia principle is linked to an informative transfer whose efficiency depends on the difference between the informative ability of the remedy given by the physician compared to the patient.

The paradigm of signifiers therefore opens up a new possibility in the exploration of informative therapeutics. Since the beginning of Life, interrelationships between the first organisms and their environment progressively allowed all structures to interact. The different levels of information have organized the spread of signifiers, each level being the regulation and integration of the previous one in an integrative hierarchy. The living self is the never-ending process whereby levels of information are synthesized, in the face of the informing environment.

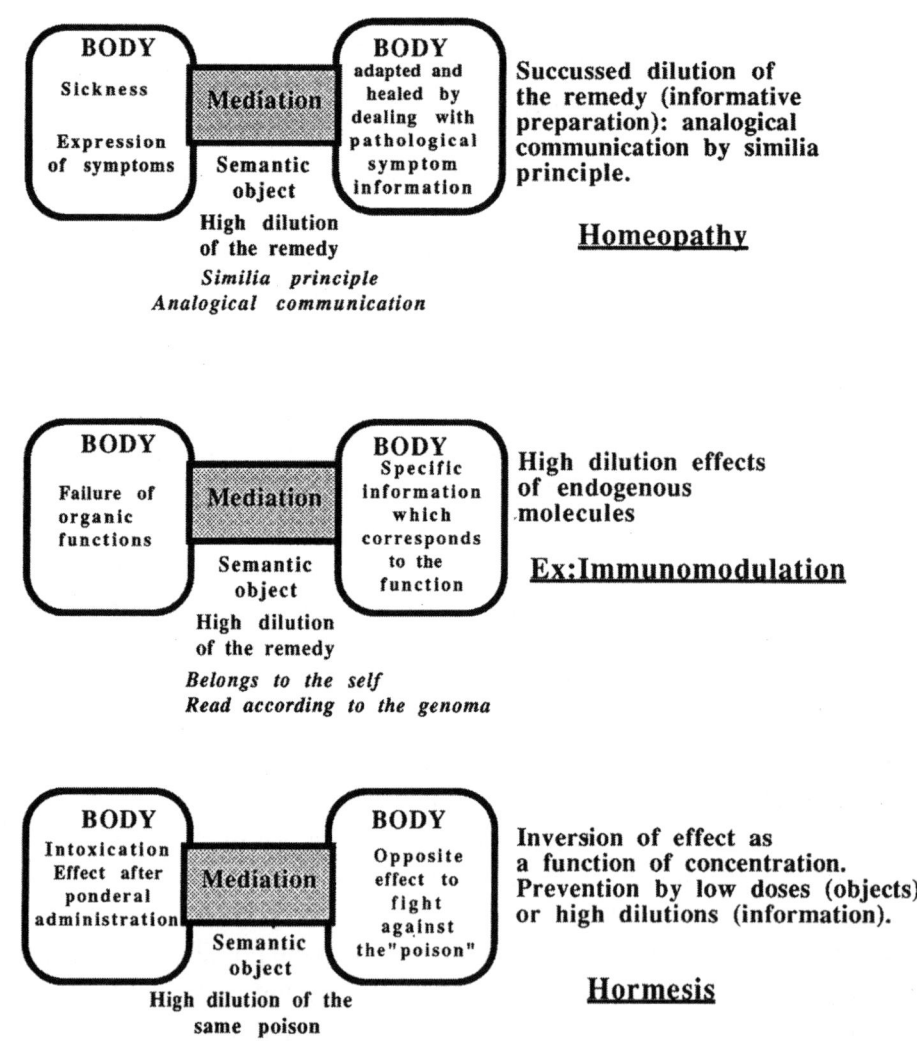

Figure 5: High dilution effect interpretation in the paradigm of signifiers

References

Aldridge, D.
1989 "Music, communication and medicine: discussion paper", in: *J. Royal Soc. Med.*, 82: 743-746.
1993 "Music and Alzheimer disease-assessment and therapy: discussion paper", in: *J. Royal Soc. Med.*, 86: 93-95.

Aldridge, D., Gustorff, G. and Hannich, H. J.
1990 "Music therapy applied to coma patients", in: *J. Royal Soc. Med.*, 83: 345-346.

Bastide, M.
1996a "Basic research on high dilution effects", in: C. Taddei and P. Marotta (eds.): *High Dilution Effects on Cells and Integrated Systems*, World Scientific Publ.: Singapore, New Jersey, London. *In press*.

Bastide, M. and Boudard, F.
1996b "High dilutions as a tool of immunomodulation", in: C. Taddei and P. Marotta (eds.): *High Dilution Effects on Cells and Integrated Systems*, World Scientific Publ.: Singapore, New Jersey, London. *In press*.

Bastide, M. and Lagache, A.
1992 *The Paradigm of Signifiers,* Alpha Bleue Publishers: Paris.
1996 "A new paradigm applied to high dilution effects on the living body", in: C. Taddei and P. Marotta (eds.): *High Dilution Effects on Cells and Integrated Systems*, World Scientific Publ.: Singapore, New Jersey, London. *In press*.

Bastide, M., Lagache, A. and Lemaire-Misonne, C.
1995 "Le paradigme des signifiants: schème d'information applicable à l'Immunologie et à l'Homéopathie", in: *Revue Intern. Systémique*, 9: 237-249.

Bateson, G.
1977 *Steps to an Ecology of Mind*, Chandler Publisher: New York.

Delbancut, A.
1994 "Contribution à l'étude des effets de hautes dilutions de métaux vis-à-vis de la cytotoxicité du Cadmium sur des cultures de cellules tubulaires rénales", in: *Thèse Université Bordeaux II, France*, Juillet 1994.

Doutremepuich, C., Aguejouf, O., Pintigny, D., Sertillanges, N. M. and De Seze, O.
1994 "Thrombogenic properties of ultra-low-doses of acetylsalicylic acid in a vessel model of laser-induced thrombus formation", in: *Thrombosis Research*, 76: 225-229.

Endler, P. C., Pongratz, W., Kastberger, G., Wiegant, F. A. C. and Schulte, J.
1994 "The effect of highly diluted agitated thyroxine on the climbing activity of frogs", in:*Vet. Hum. Tox.*, 36: 56-59.

Hadji, L., Arnoux, B. and Benveniste, J.
1992 "Effect of dilute histamine on coronary flow of guinea-pig isolated heart. Inhibition by a magnetic field", in: *FASEB*, no.7040.

Lagache, A.
1988   *Echos du Sensible*, Alpha Bleue Publisher: Paris.
1996a   "Notes on the conceptual basis of Science", in: M. Bastide (ed.): *Signal and Images*, Kluwer Academic Publisher: Dordrecht. *In press*.
1996b   "What is Information", in: M. Bastide (ed.): *Signal and Images*, Kluwer Academic Publisher: Dordrecht. *In press*.

Oberbaum, M. and Cambar, J.
1994   "Hormesis; dose dependent reverse effects of low and very low doses", in: Endler and Schulte (eds.): *Ultra High Dilution, Physiology and Physics,* pp. 5-19, Kluwer Academic Publisher: Dordrecht.

Van Wijk, R., Welters, M., Souren, J. A., Ovelgonne, H. and Wiegant, F. A. C.
1993   "Serum-stimulated cell cycle progression and stress protein synthesis in C3H10T1/2 fibroblasts treated with sodium arsenite", in: *J. Cell. Physiology*, 155: 265-272.

Van Wijk,R.,Ooms,H.,Wiegant,F.A.C.,Souren,J.E.M.,Ovelgönne,J.H.,van Aken,J.M. and Bol,A.W.J.M.
1994   "A molecular basis for understanding the benefits from subharmful doses of toxicants; an experimental approach to the concepts of hormesis and the homeopathic similia law", in:*Environ. Manag. Health*, 5: 13-25.

Weis, P. and Weis, J. S.
1986   "Cadmium acclimation and hormesis in Fundulus heteroclitus during fin regeneration", in: *Environ. Res.*, 39: 356-363.

Youbicier-Simo, B. J., Boudard, F., Mekaouche, M., Bastide, M. and Baylé, J. D.
1993   "Effects of embryonic bursectomy and *in ovo* administration of highly diluted bursin on adrenocorticotropic and immune response of chickens", in: *Int. J. Immunotherapy,* 9: 169-180.

Part II

Medical Pluralism

The Polyglot Practitioner: Towards Acceptance of Different Approaches in Treatment Evaluation

by Elisabeth Hsu

"Therapeutic efficacy" is currently one of the main criteria for the legitimisation of alternative medicines in European health care. The therapeutic efficacy of a certain treatment is mostly assessed by randomised double blind-tests where a "placebo" treatment is given to members of a control group. Among many professionals of the biomedical establishment, and within them large parts of the public, it is still considered the sole method that is scientifically reliable and has general validity. As desirable as a quantitative assessment of "therapeutic efficacy" may be, it poses serious problems if taken as sole criterium for treatment evaluation (e.g., Lewith & Aldridge 1993).[1]

This paper will first recall historical evidence that questions the assumption that it was the "efficacy" of biomedical treatments that led to their acceptance, which in turn questions the current imperative to assess "therapeutic efficacy" of alternative treatments. The importance that the biomedical establishment attributes to biomedically assessed "efficacy" is probably best understood as a means to exert control over medical knowledge. "Therapeutic efficacy" is closely associated with the biomedical conception of "disease", a concept that has high validity within biomedical practice, but is hardly useful for understanding the therapeutic considerations and interventions of alternative practitioners. Nor does it help to understand the patient's experiences, and it has some in-built limitations for the biomedically trained doctor too.

The paper will then proceed to conceptualise the frequently observed non-communication of treatment evaluation between practitioners of alternative medicines, patients and professionals of the biomedical establishment as a "language" problem. Having established that "efficacy" belongs to the "language" of biomedicine, and cannot claim general validity, possibilities for recording the

---

[1] This paper was delivered at the INRAT Seminar on "Communication in and about alternative therapies" as a contribution to the workshop on "Communication about alternative therapies in medicine and research", 29th September – 1st October 1995. I would like to thank the participants of the workshop as well as Peter Flubacher and Bruno Riek for their valuable comments on an earlier draft.

experiences of the actors of the clinical encounter are outlined. The goal is to find means for both practitioners and patients to express their evaluation of the treatment as faithfully as possible in their own language. I suggest making a basic distinction between the patient's evaluation that accounts for "therapeutic quality" and the intervening practitioner's evaluation of "therapeutic results," irrespective of whether the treatment is alternative or biomedical.

Since the actors' understanding of one and the same treatment can differ greatly and be difficult to bring into accordance (Lewis 1993), the paper, thirdly, will provide some case material to show possibilities of how a social scientist may help (or not help) in evaluating the different perspectives and thereby contribute to treatment evaluation. In this connection, I will define the notion of "therapeutic success" as one that takes account of socially relevant events, personal and cultural meanings attributed to them, and their interdependence with economic and political circumstances. As will be shown, the "therapeutic success" and the "therapeutic efficacy" of a treatment need not always coincide, whereas they may mutually condition each other (cf. table 1).

Table 1: Different approaches towards treatment evaluation

the evaluators' position	their conceptual framework	aspect of treatment evaluation
the actors:		
the patient	own body and self	"therapeutic quality"
the practitioner	the alternative medicine or biomedicine	"therapeutic results"
the observers:		
the biomedical scientist	biomedical subdisciplines, epidemiology, statistics, etc.	"therapeutic efficacy"
the social scientist	the social sciences, e.g., medical anthropology	"therapeutic success"

"Therapeutic Efficacy" in Historical Perspective

The myth of modern science and medicine as a series of discoveries generating a never-ending progress has been sufficiently deconstructed; historical evidence need not be reiterated here. This is said without wanting to belittle the researchers whose unremitting efforts – and sometimes personal sacrifice – led to these achievements. However, Copernicus' findings did not allow for as precise calculations as Ptolemaic astronomy did (Kuhn 1976: 88); Wassermann's test for syphilis was in its first applications misinterpreted (Fleck 1994: 94); antisepsis was hardly more effective than alternative procedures, and vaccine therapy, which is nowadays regarded as a failure, persisted, at least for chronic conditions, until displaced by antibiotics (Pickstone 1992: 15). The sociology and history of science and medicine has shown that scientific and medical practices were often endorsed or relinquished independently of their "efficacy".

Even if the history of medicine reveals that "efficacy" was not as important as generally believed, current efforts directed at the goal of assessing "efficacy" are perfectly legitimate to the medical professional and anyone who supports the hegemony of biomedicine. It needs to be kept in mind, however, that the achievements that have led to the now well-established biomedicine were made within a conceptual framework that set certain priorities. The focus on material and static entities as in anatomy, localisation of function in substance as in pathophysiology/histology, identification of pathogen as in bacteriology, materialisation of therapeutic agency as in the pharmaceutica – insulin, sulfonamids, antibiotics, etc. – has led to a validation of quantity over quality, of matter over the spiritual, of visibly enduring entities over rhythmically returning ones. This leaves a view of the person reduced to a body, an assessment of sickness reduced to disease entities, an understanding of therapy reduced to method. Randomised double-blind tests and the notion of "therapeutic efficacy" build on such premises. "Therapeutic efficacy" is treatment, method, and substance-oriented; it accounts for a standardised, itemised, and time-limited therapeutic intervention.

Historians have shown that specific medical interventions alone did not lead to the decline of morbidity (e.g., McKeown 1976). Infectious diseases were not reduced by antibiotics alone, but largely by economic and social circumstances that increased hygiene. Tuberculosis morbidity declined before the advent of chemotherapy, due to elimination of malnutrition and overcrowding. Living conditions, environmental factors like air, water or noise pollution, nutrition, mental and emotional nurturance, attitudes to self and other, habits and daily activities – in short, the "style of life" plays a prominent role in preventive as well as curative health care.

From a historical perspective, the general acceptance of a medical practice sometimes happened quite independently of its efficacy. "Therapeutic efficacy" is a notion that emerged on the basis of a very specific understanding of personhood and well-being. It is a concept, like any other concept, that has its strengths and limitations. It should not be seen as universal, but as useful in a defined context of application. Therapeutic efficacy belongs to the means I advocate for evaluating treatment from an observer's perspective in section three. However, before embarking on that discussion, let us take account of how the actors of the clinical encounter themselves evaluate treatment.

The Actors' Perspectives:
"Therapeutic Quality" and "Therapeutic Results"

Research in alternative medicine has outlined some methods for evaluating treatment which have great significance because they empower the actors. Some of those methods are explicitly directed at evaluating the quality of the treatment from the patient's viewpoint. Others record the alternative practitioners' perceptions, their conceptualisation of the patient's condition, their calculations, and the results of their intervention.

Experience and the patient's evaluation of treatment: "Therapeutic Quality"
Assessments of the "quality of life" (QoL) generally belong among the more formalised approaches for recording a patient's subjective experiences. Since they allow for a certain operationalisation of the patient's perspective, they have attracted the attention of many biomedically trained physicians. The need to consider the patient as a person arose largely in the context of cancer treatment and chemotherapy, where the side-effects of a treatment often were dehumanising and the prolongation of life was opposed to an improvement of the quality of life (Fallowfield 1990). QoL tests and questionnaires are innumerable; they are grounded in many different theoretical traditions, with the concept itself often defined in a very narrow way. A definition of the QoL that is explicitly designed to account for individual experience and the processual aspects of treatment evaluation: *"QoL is what the patient says it is, his or her own response to the match between individual desire or intention, on the one hand, and performance and capacity on the other"* (Joyce 1991: 14). As general as such a concept may appear, it is ultimately thought to provide a quantitative assessment of quality.

"Single case studies", first used in circles of experimental psychology and psychoanalysis, have the advantage of recording the patient's viewpoint in a more extensive and less formalised way. Diary recording deserves particular attention here. It has been shown to have the advantage of providing a comprehensive view of the patient's perceptions of symptoms "as episodes", i.e., as *"diffuse conditions which may not be disabling or necessitate intervention but which contribute to the profile of the patient's symptomatology."* Moreover, it accounts for the patient's relational context, subjective feelings and experiences. The drawbacks are that they reflect the patient's "bias" (which is not surprising since patients are supposed to express their subjective feelings) and, more importantly, that the wealth of information cannot be processed in a systematic way. One cannot intend to make a statement of general validity (Aldridge 1993).

"Illness narratives" could be used as yet another means for evaluating treatment. In anthropology, they have mostly been used as research data. Kleinman (1988) has set an example for recording the patient's subjective interpretation of illness, whereby special attention is drawn to social and cultural aspects of individual experience. As Steffen (1995) points out, *"illness accounts can also be told by lay person to lay person without any reference to scientific interpretations as happens all the time in therapeutic groups like Alcoholics Anonymous."* Life story telling is a process central to human experience, and shared experience has proved therapeutic. The reason I mention "illness narratives" in this context is that they appear to provide keys for understanding a patient's perception and evaluation of the treatment.

Case records and the intervening practitioner's evaluation of treatment: the "Therapeutic Results"

Medical practitioners generally engage in case recording. This is nothing new. Case records provide not only useful evidence in a law suit, but more importantly, they are a heuristic device. The information accumulated in case records is used for diagnostics as well as therapeutics, and, in the end, also as a means for evaluating the outcome of a treatment. Case records nicely reflect the ways in which a medical practitioner conceptualises the problems of a client, what she perceives as important, which aspects of the client's disablement she decides to treat, and how she evaluates the therapeutic intervention.

I propose to view case records as recording information on the "result" of a therapy. I speak of "results" because, like results in mathematics, "therapeutic results" report on a series of calculations. Like results of calculations, the information they convey needs to be sensibly interpreted for an evaluation of what they describe – observations from case records can be misleading (e.g., Schmidt 1994).

"Therapeutic results" are invaluable for treatment evaluation, not only because they provide an actor's point of view, but also because they provide information on specialised knowledge about the treatment. It seems important to me that therapeutic results are recorded as consistently as possible in terms of the framework within which a practitioner operates. In other words, if a practitioner is "polyglot" and can think both in terms of biomedicine and alternative medicine, rather than opting for a so-called "trajective discourse" (see below), the results should be separately recorded in each "language".

Crucial for biomedical diagnosis is depersonalisation; case records are thus depersonalised. After taking up the data of a person – name, age, sex, address, insurance number etc. – the information considered relevant for medical treatment is noted separately. This separation of the biological processes from the person is necessary because biomedicine aims at identifying disease entities that basically have the same etiology, pathogenesis, symptomatology, and can be treated with basically the same therapeutic means. Needless to say, the identification of disease entities is one of the major achievements of the biomedical sciences. The depersonalised view of patients has, however, serious drawbacks,[2] particularly if one is faced with psychosomatic and chronic conditions as most practitioners in alternative medicines are.

Oliver Sacks, in recognition of this problem, speaks in his book *Awakenings* of the method of "trajective discourse", a style of recording case histories where the doctor views himself as a traveller into the world of illness. "Trajective discourse" conforms to what the anthropologist Clifford Geertz calls "thick description". It is, like thick description, contextually grounded: *"It emphasizes as relevant to a patient history a sense of character, life-history, important human relationships (with both family and staff), and personal values and goals of the individual patient"* (Hunsaker Hawkins 1993). Neither the doctor's nor the patient's subjective impressions are effaced. Trajective discourse integrates intersubjective biomedical findings with the subjective and personal views (of doctor and patient) in one and the same paragraph. Sacks elegantly blends the Latin of biomedicine and the English of a traveller in the world of illness into one language, the poetics of trajective discourse.

Lesser mortals may find it difficult to imitate his art of writing in daily medical practice. For pragmatic reasons, I therefore propose, as a more viable means of evaluating a therapeutic intervention, to record "therapeutic results" in terms of the medical framework within which an alternative practitioner operates. It is important for alternative practitioners to stick to their "language" and record the events as consistently as possible in terms of the alternative medicine.

---

[2] Anspach (1988) found that case presentations in various biomedical establishments had the following traits in common: 1. depersonalisation, i.e., the separation of the biological processes from the person, 2. use of the passive voice, i.e., omission of the agent, 3. medical technology is used as an agent, 4. account markers such as "states", "reports", "denies", etc. emphasize the subjectivity of the client's account.

The Observers' Perspective:
"Therapeutic Efficacy" and "Therapeutic Success"

As already said above, the biomedical assessment of "therapeutic efficacy" belongs to the chief methods for assessing any medical treatment, regardless of whether it is conventional or unconventional. It is important that the "efficacy" of treatment be evaluated by an *observer* who is well-informed and sensitised to the difficulties of assessing it.[3] The biomedical assessment of therapeutic efficacy is by no means straightforward. Discussions often arise as to which parameters are to be considered significant, when the measurements are best to be taken, which factors can produce misleading results, which size of the samples allows for a statement of reasonable validity, which statistics are to be applied etc. This is said to point to the complexities involved in assessing therapeutic efficacy – both in biomedicine and alternative medicine – and explain why treatment evaluation by means of therapeutic efficacy has to be endorsed with care.

Another approach towards evaluating treatment, put forth in the following, is the assessment of so-called "therapeutic success". The distinction that I propose to make between "therapeutic efficacy" and "therapeutic success" draws on Kleinman's (1980) distinction between "disease" and "illness". "Disease" is nowadays understood to refer to a person's pathological condition in terms of biomedicine. "Illness" refers to the patient's and her surrounding's subjective experience of distress and etiology, and furthermore to the general way in which the disablement is perceived in the patient's social context.[4] "Therapeutic efficacy" would thus account for the treatment of a patient's disease, "therapeutic success" of the patient's illness.

Disease and illness
Research in medical anthropology has shown how far-reaching consequences the view of the social environment and the cultural construction of illness can have. One of the most striking findings is that in some cases the diseased are con-

---

[3] This means that even if the intervening practitioners of an alternative medicine are biomedically trained, they themselves cannot assess the "therapeutic efficacy" because they belong among the actors of the clinical encounter.

[4] Eisenberg (1977: 9) distinguished "disease" from "illness" as professional versus popular ideas of sickness: *"The patients suffer 'illnesses'; the doctors [traditional healers included] diagnose and treat 'diseases'."* Kleinman (1980) modified the terms with the result that nowadays "disease" is generally understood to refer to the biomedical assessment of dysfunction and "illness" to a cultural construction (that is not biomedical). Young (1982) criticised these two psychiatrists' approach because it neglected to view sickness as a social phenomenon and underplayed the political interests involved in the process of determining and overcoming it.

sidered "normal" while those who are, according to biomedicine, healthy are excluded from social interaction: In Southern Argentina, there was apparently a group of people who were all infected by a fungus which "decorated" the skin (*dichromic spirochaetosis*). Those not infected were not allowed to marry (Ackerknecht 1947). Even a disease like measles with high fever and skin rashes can be regarded as a "normal" stage of growing. Chinese mothers consider it to be caused by *taidu*, the womb's poison, that has to be washed out of the body, and they take it as a necessary stage of child development (Topley 1968).

More often, however, the phenomenon that biomedicine diagnoses as disease is also recognised by peoples in other societies as illness. The difference lies in the ways in which this reality is reinterpreted. Among the Gnau in New Guinea, a man who has insulted the ancestors (a social deviance) may find that he suffers from shivers and high fever (a physical disturbance that can be biomedically assessed, but does not primarily arise from an organic dysfunction); he will disrupt all social interaction, and retire into the dark and dust of a little hut to recover from his illness. Or, a woman who suffers from wasting muscles may attribute this to the anger of a spirit, while a biomedic recognises a serious neurological disease (Lewis 1976). Since she continues to participate in daily life, she may call her legs "rotten" (*wola*), and not refer to herself as "ill" (*neyigeg*).

Sometimes, however, a non-disease like the discharge of women is considered an illness, as in the case of Korean women suffering from *naeng*, coldness (Sich 1978). Although no bacteria, not even thrush is found in the discharge, and although the gynaecologist explains that discharge can increase in situations of stress and sometimes also for no apparent reason (Harrison's 1988: 512), this discharge has a social reality that can jeopardize a young woman's fate: Her dowry may be reduced or, even worse, she may be taken off the marriage market altogether.

One may consider it futile to compare and contrast incidences of illness with their reinterpretation in terms of biomedicine as disease. It was done above to show that in many contexts, the biomedical assessment of disease is irrelevant to what constitutes an illness, to what determines a person's behaviour, social interaction, and day-to-day life. Kleinman (1980: 82) made a distinction between the "curing of disease" and the "healing of illness". Healing reasserted threatened values and arbitrated social tensions; curing removed bodily symptoms. He emphasized that the resolution of social tensions was often the primary target of a healer.

In consideration of the frequent discrepancy between the dynamics of what members of a society consider an illness and what a doctor diagnoses as disease, the distinction between "therapeutic efficacy" and "therapeutic success" is made in a similar vein.⁵ "Therapeutic efficacy" would then refer to the effects of a therapy that biomedicine can measure and assess, "therapeutic success" to what the patients and their social environment consider the success of the treatment. The reason I speak of "success" is because success clearly has to do with social dynamics, often regardless of quality. Moreover, the wording "therapeutic success" has already been used in a similar way by researchers of alternative medicines (Anthony & Parsons 1993: 47ff, Aldridge 1993: 137).

The evaluation of "therapeutic success" requires research that is quite distinct from the investigation of therapeutic efficacy. Although the term "therapeutic success" has so far not been used in the anthropological literature, descriptions that amount to a circumscribing of this phenomenon abound. One of the most frequently mentioned achievements of traditional and unconventional healers has been shown to arise from their reinterpretation of the patient's condition. Time is too limited to give a comprehensive summary of ways in which the reinterpretation of an illness can result in therapeutic success or failure that does not coincide with its biomedical assessment. The following two examples merely highlight two possibilities.

One example shows that a therapeutic intervention like *qigong* healing can be successful in so far as it leads to an alteration of a patient's subjective perception of his/her condition, whereby little has changed from a biomedical point of view (i.e., the therapeutic efficacy was minimal). The other example demonstrates how a healer's reinterpretation can lead to the patient's compliance and cooperation that may eventually result in behaviour leading to recovery (i.e., maximum therapeutic efficacy). Both examples concern a *qigong* healer in the People's Republic of China who had a family practice in a populous area of Kunming city.⁶

---

5   Notice that the "healing of illness" refers to values and social tensions and the "curing of disease" concerns bodily symptoms in Kleinman (1980). This distinction may trigger the misunderstanding that healers heal and biomedics cure which is simply wrong. The distinction I make is grounded in the professional training of the observer and the means by which the information is obtained: biomedically trained doctors can diagnose disease and assess therapeutic efficacy; social scientists are trained to account for the cultural construction of illness and assess therapeutic success. The difference is fine, but relevant.

6   In the West, *qigong* (discipline of the breath) has become known mostly as a meditative practice. It may be practised as daily meditation to the effect of longevity, but it is also known for its therapeutic success. An individual may want to meditate alone or in groups; she may stand, sit or lie on the floor; there are different exercises and breathing techniques. *Qigong* is not a standardised therapy and there are just as many forms of *qigong* as there are masters. In the People's Republic of China an even larger range of different practices are called *qigong*. They range from marvel-invoking spectacles at market fairs (fire swallowing, glass eating, bricks being slammed apart on one's head etc.) to a particular gymnastics taught at schools. The *qigong* healer I worked with engaged in activities which were directed at manipulating the energies of the patient, whereby the patient was not asked to do anything, except to sit still and close the eyes. *Qigong* healing consisted of a public session and a private one. The public

Example 1
The first case concerns a woman in her fifties who suffered from bad shoulder pain. She was a remarkable client because of her high social status (a high school teacher), her vivacious cooperation (talkative, encouraging, and easily influenced) and her persistent health-seeking behaviour. The pain in her shoulder had set in four months earlier, for no apparent reason. She first went to the most prestigious hospital of Kunming. Like so many state-educated and state-employed cadres, she turned first to biomedicine, but the doctor she consulted sent her to the acumoxa department of that hospital. She was treated for a fortnight without visible improvement. By then she had learnt that professionally trained acupuncturists worked at Chinese medical hospitals. But the treatment at the First City Chinese Medical Hospital did not prove much more successful. Her arm still hurt badly and prevented her from sleeping at night. Masseurs of an itinerant medical service group, stationed at the doorsteps of the hospital, promised a definite cure after inspecting her shoulder. For a quarter of her monthly salary, paid in advance, she was guaranteed daily treatment until her arm was cured. This treatment worsened her pain to such an extent that she could hardly lift her arm anymore. She then turned to *qigong*.

The director of a private *qigong* hospital,[7] who was the said healer's bond brother, recommended him to her. When the healer heard that his bond brother had refused to treat her, he expressed doubts as well. She was, however, anxious to receive his treatment and pointed out that he had just cured a patient in front of her eyes in one single session. *"Everyone is different,"* he replied. *"For qigong you've got to have 'predestined fate' (yuanfen)."*[8] He eventually agreed to give it a try. In addition to acumoxa, cupping jar, fire massage[9] and *qigong* treatment, he proposed to deliver *yuan-qigong* (far-away-effect *qigong*) which he and his disciple would send in the evenings from their home to her's on the other

---

    one was an almost theatrical performance which comprised movements with which the healer extracted the bad *qi* from the patient and others for transmitting his original *qi*, thereby invigorating the patient. The private one was meditative in which the healer restored his own energies. For a detailed discussion of this healer's *qigong* cf. Hsu 1992, chapters 3-4.

7   There are *qigong* hospitals in the PRC where *qigong* healers work in a professionalised setting. The *qigong* hospital in Kunming was set up by a son of a high official who was given much credit by the banks, but it went bankrupt after half a year.

8   This seems to be a general rule for alternative medicines. The reason is not that the "method" is unreliable, but that the understanding of what a human being is, differs radically from that of biomedicine.

9   The bottom of a jar is covered with a medicinal alcohol which is saturated with the ingredients of several herbal medicines. With a piece of burning cotton stuck onto scissors, the alcohol is lit and put onto the patient's sore places with the therapeut's left hand. His right hand, with which he delivers massage, suffocates the flame and rubs the alcohol into the skin. This method, which I observed to kill pain and reduce swellings effectively, is not practised in government hospitals; the said *qigong* healer commented: "It is very hard work."

side of the city. *Yuan-qigong* consisted of the simultaneous "meditation in tranquility" (*jinggong*) of sender and receiver.

The treatment that followed comprised about eight sessions over a period of two weeks, sessions that usually took place inside the healer's practice, except one that took place late at night, outside in the dark of a park, and the one that was held in the client's home – and turned out to be the last one. It was held on a Sunday afternoon, after the client had prepared a most elaborate meal for the healer, his wife, the healer's disciple and the anthropologist. After the rich banquet and an afternoon stroll along the lake, the client asked to be treated. The healer had not expected this. He was not in the mood and felt tired. Instead, he had his disciple deliver *qigong*. It was the first time that the disciple was to perform a session without his master. An hour of silence followed while the disciple was with the client in a separate room. As the silence persisted, the healer eventually went to check what was happening. When he opened the door, the patient broke out into enthusiastic exclamations: She had felt a tingling in the arm going right up to the shoulder! To everyone's surprise, the disciple had had a key experience during this session and thereby acquired a cognitive faculty that is basic to delivering the *qigong* therapy he was being trained in. Our entire group, the healer, his wife, the client, her husband and I started clapping our hands and dancing and shouting and being very excited about the disciple's achievement.

After this moving incident, the client required no more treatment, and only came to pay the fee, a sum that exceeded her monthly salary. She could lift her shoulder only a few degrees higher, but she claimed to be much better. More than that, when I spoke to her a year later, I learnt that she had not sought treatment with other healers anymore. Her work unit had not had any further expenses for endless treatments. Despite an improvement that was from a biomedical point of view only one of degree – the therapeutic efficacy of the treatment was practically nil – her behaviour changed drastically, from that of an ill to that of a healthy person. In this respect, the healer and his disciple could rightly claim that their therapy had been most successful.

You may say, well, it was not the "method" of a *qigong* performance and its rationale that made the therapy successful; it was the excitement, the healer's devotion, and all the emotional upheaval in the end. Ritual intervention is an event that always involves the senses – with odours, aromas, heat, colours, rhythm, and music – and triggers off emotions – fear, joy, anger, sorrow, and awe. That it can lead to therapeutic success is amply recorded in the anthropological literature. Even if from a biomedical point of view the therapeutic efficacy of *qigong* might be minimal, the altered social behaviour following such ritual performance is just as important, if not more important for the person who was declared or declared herself ill.

Example 2
The following example shows that a reinterpretation of a patient's condition can also happen in a rationally more intelligible way. Again, the healer's main target was to alter the patient's perception of self, and accordingly her behaviour. Chronic ailments and psychosomatic syndromes which tend to be the main complaints unconventional healing methods are applied to, are not cured overnight. Nor do they always disappear completely. If the patient can comply with the healer, therapeutic success is not far away, and the therapy may prove to be biomedically efficacious, as will be shown below.

The *qigong* healer's main achievement in the case recorded here was that his reinterpretation, in terms of Chinese medical reasoning, built on the same values as his client's did in everyday life, values that do not necessarily conform to biomedical ones.

> "When I arrived at the *qigong* practice, the healer was massaging a young woman. He refused to give me any explanations, yet she readily talked to me. She had had an abortion four months ago. That was when it all started. At the hospital, she was diagnosed as suffering from neurasthenia *(shenjing shuairuo)*. 'This is wrong', she said and explained that the *qigong* healer had given her the correct diagnosis: 'Blood Depletion giving rise to Wind *(xue xu sheng feng)* which induced dizziness and headaches'. She had been in treatment for five days now, a combined treatment of massage, herbal medicines, and *qigong*. Did she feel any better? Yes, but she now felt like vomiting *(xiang tu)*. She added she only had a headache now when she felt unhappy and angry.

> "Why did she have an abortion in the fifth month? Her answer was that she had stomach problems and took lots of medicine in alcohol. Her sister, who was a doctor, said her child would be mentally retarded, so she aborted it. After the abortion, she did not 'go into confinement' *(zuo yuezi)*, she said.

> "'To disregard confinement is a typical case for Blood Depletion giving rise to Wind', the healer's wife commented. 'She went shopping and she did not even cover her head!' She meant that this client had exposed herself to the wind in the streets and thereby attracted the Wind in her head which induced the headache. She spoke in terms of common knowledge (reasoning reminiscent of sympathetic magic). Chinese medical reasoning is more sophisticated: headaches (symptoms) are often associated with Wind (a postulated process), Wind that ascends to the head when

there is a Blood Depletion (a postulated process that is an Inner Disease Factor *(neiyin)*). Needless to say, the blood lost during the abortion had caused the Blood Depletion inside the body" (notes, 8th August 1989).

The healer later explained to me that this client had been divorced by her husband and aborted the child thereafter. He showed much affection for this young woman, and his wife who noticed this too, was eager to have him terminate treatment soon.[10]

The reinterpretation in Chinese medical terms fitted very well into the client's world view and reinforced her values. First, the *qigong* healer made the nonobservance of confinement responsible for her suffering. Confinement after birth (traditionally for forty days) is currently advocated even among Chinese biomedical doctors, and women doctors practise it themselves. This client explained that she had never thought of confinement after an abortion. I had not heard about such a rule either, but the healer's decision to make use of the flexibility of this rule and apply it to this particular case was certainly appropriate: The client's experience of the abortion had not been a scratching out of some bloody stuff (as it is in the first three months of a pregnancy), but a birth, albeit of a dead foetus. Going into confinement meant that someone had to cook and care for her. She had missed out on this. No allowances had been made towards her pain and suffering. The healer's reinterpretation of the situation allowed her to take a break and rest.

Second, she easily could relate to the healer's statement that she suffered from a so-called Blood Depletion. Naturally, Blood Depletion (*xue xu*), as a technical Chinese medical term, was not directly intelligible to her. She simply understood that it referred to a loss of blood, the blood she herself had seen flowing. This is an important characteristic of indigenous medicines. The specialised medical terms are the same words as those of everyday language, but their meaning is not quite the same.

Xue in Chinese medicine does refer to the blood that the patient had seen flowing, but it is also an abstract term within a system of similarly abstract terms (e.g., *qi* energies, *jing* essences, *shen* spirits). Blood Depletion referred to a state of the person that could be identified by particular diagnostic signs like a white face, a thin pulse, a pale tongue etc. Blood Depletions can be diagnosed even if the patient has not suffered from an obvious blood loss. According to Chinese

---

10 I hesitate to condemn this personal involvement of the healer with his client as immoral, although he went to the limits of what is morally acceptable for a married man in China. Is such personal involvement and empathy of the healer with difficult clients not a "method" characteristic of some alternative medicines?

medical reasoning, a "distinguishing pattern", like a Blood Depletion, does not contain any information on the etiology of the condition (see also Farquhar 1994: 86-91, Hsu forthcoming). Rather, it is a therapeutic maxim: If a doctor "diagnoses" a Blood Depletion, this means that the therapy should be directed at restoring the Blood.

The treatment of Blood Depletions also made sense to the client: It was common knowledge among Chinese laypersons that a diet of eggs (vitality bolstering), meat (particularly liver and fish), 'red' sugar (the sugar actually looks brown, but by calling it 'red', it was associated with happiness and wealth, and in medical terms with enlivening *yang* qualities). This would restore her Blood. She also drank the Blood-restoring drug potions the healer had prescribed, even if they were very bitter (*tai ku liao*). The diet was pleasant and brought colour into her face; the medication was aimed at restoring her own energies and visibly enhanced her drive for activity. What a contrast to the anti-depressives that she had been previously prescribed.

The healer not only provided her with a verbal reinterpretation of her condition, his treatment was also directed at relieving her bodily symptoms.[11] He delivered massage (on the head) if she complained of headaches, or he laid his hand onto her belly for *qigong* if she felt like vomiting. Moreover, he wanted her to actively engage in her recovery and taught her movements to practise *qigong* on her own. She said she practised *qigong* in the evenings at home before going to sleep; it cleared her mind. Last but not least, the healer was someone who always retained his cheerfulness (*kailang*) – which is, among Chinese people, held in high esteem as a quality of Taoist adepts. Moreover, his personal sympathy for her obviously lifted her spirits. After about two months of treatment, she seems to have been driven away by the healer's wife, but in a visibly better state of health – she had joined the working force again.

Reinterpretations of an ailment not only restructure client's illness experience, but are also a means to gain their compliance and engage them actively in their therapy. In this case, the therapeutic success of the entire treatment could have been assessed in terms of therapeutic efficacy as well. It would have been difficult to evaluate, however, the efficacy of each of the "methods" and "substances" the *qigong* healer delivered.

---

11 In Kleinman's (1980) terminology, this healer "healed" and "cured" the patient.

Summary

The two examples from the *qigong* healer's practice in China show that therapeutic interventions should not be assessed with regard to "therapeutic efficacy" alone. "Therapeutic efficacy" may well evaluate the effectiveness of a therapy with regard to "disease" in a standardised and quantitative way, but this information is not sufficient for evaluating the well-being of a person and her reintegration into her social environment.

"Therapeutic success" provides an assessment of the treatment in view of the client's "illness" and the experienced personal, social, and cultural dimensions of her condition. In these two cases, I may not have sufficiently taken account of the economic aspect of the chronic ailments for the individual as well as for the society at large. Since the accounts were written in non-standardised ways, one can easily imagine an assessment of "therapeutic success" that considers these factors as well. Deliberately, no attempt was made to formalise the levels and dimensions of these cases, which leaves more space to account for the interdependencies of the relevant aspects for evaluating illness. This approach contests that only numbers can provide the necessary clarity for evaluating treatment, and can highlight aspects of the treatment that escape the assessment of "therapeutic efficacy".

As outlined in the beginning, treatment cannot be evaluated without considering the actors involved, namely the patients and practitioners. The "therapeutic results" that the alternative practitioner records often contain information grounded in specialised knowledge that neither a natural nor a social scientist has learned to perceive. Even if the language of the practitioner appears strange, it should not be dismissed from the very start. Since the goal of any treatment is to improve the condition of the clients, it would be truly foolish to disregard their subjective experience and the evaluation of treatment, the "therapeutic quality".

The evaluation of alternative medicines poses interesting epistemological problems. There are different modalities of perception, different attitudes to what constitutes evidence, and different "languages" to account for it. This paper encourages research that evaluates treatment from different angles. Treatment evaluation that requires interdisciplinary research groups certainly does more justice to the situation, while it cannot guarantee any consensus in the end. However, if actors and observers, perfectly entitled as they are to speak their own "language", refuse to make an effort to understand the others', not even communication, let alone consensus, about alternative therapies can succeed.

References

Ackerknecht, Erwin W.
1947   "The Role of Medical History in Medical Education", in: *Bulletin of the History of Medicine*, 21: 135-145.

Aldridge, David
1993   "Single Case Research Design", in: G.T. Lewith & D. Aldridge (eds.): *Clinical Research Methodology for Complementary Therapies*, pp. 136-168, Hodder & Stoughton: London.

Anthony, Honor M. & Parsons, Frank M.
1993   "Why Measure Outcomes?", in: G.T. Lewith & D. Aldridge (eds.): *Clinical Research Methodology for Complementary Therapies*, pp. 46-56, Hodder & Stoughton: London.

Anspach R. R.
1988   "Notes on the Sociology of Medical Discourse: The Language of Case Presentation", in: J. Colombotos (ed.): *Continuities in the Sociology of Medicine. Journal of Health and Behavior*, 29: 357-375.

Eisenberg, Leon
1977   "Disease and Illness. Distinctions between Professional and Popular Ideas of Sickness", in: *Culture, Medicine and Psychiatry*, 1: 9-33.

Fallowfield, Lesley
1990   *The Quality of Life. The Missing Measurement in Health Care*, Souvenir Press: London.

Farquhar, Judith
1994   *Knowing Practice. The Clinical Encounter of Chinese Medicine*, Westview Press: Boulder.

Fleck, Ludwik
1994   *Entstehung und Entwicklung einer wissenschaftlichen Tatsache. Einführung in die Lehre vom Denkstil und Denkkollektiv*, Suhrkamp: Frankfurt a.M. (1935).

Harrison's
1988   *Harrison's Principles of Internal Medicine*, 11th edition, New York: McGraw Hill.

Hsu, Elisabeth
1992   *Transmission of Knowledge, Texts, and Treatment in Chinese Medicine*, Ph.D. in Social Anthropology, University of Cambridge.
forthc.   "Contesting Causality: 'Western Medicine treats the Symptoms, Chinese Medicine treats the Cause'", in: B.J. Andrews & A. Cunningham (eds.): *Contested Knowledge. Reactions to Western Medicine in the Modern Period*, Manchester University Press: Manchester.

Hunsaker Hawkins, Anne
1993   "Oliver Sacks' *Awakenings*: Reshaping Clinical Discourse", in: *Configurations*, 1(2): 229-245.

Joyce C. R. B.
1991   "Entwicklung der Lebensqualität in der Medizin", in: R. Schwarz et al. (eds.): *Lebensqualität in der Onkologie. Aktuelle Onkologie*, 63, 11-22. W. Zuckschwerdt: München.

Kleinman, Arthur
1980 *Patients and Healers in the Context of Culture. An Exploration of the Borderland between Anthropology, Medicine, and Psychiatry*, California University Press: Berkeley.
1988 *The Illness Narratives. Suffering, Healing, and the Human Condition*, Basic Books: New York.

Kuhn, Thomas S.
1976 *Die Struktur wissenschaftlicher Revolutionen*, Suhrkamp: Frankfurt a.M. (1962).

Lewis, Gilbert
1976 "A View of Sickness in New Guinea", in: J.B. Loudon (ed.): *Social Anthropology and Medicine*, pp. 49-103, Academic Press: London.
1993 "Double Standards of Treatment Evaluation", in: S. Lindenbaum & M. Lock (eds.): *Knowledge, Power, and Practice. The Anthropology of Medicine and Everyday Life*, pp. 189-218, University of California Press: Berkeley.

Lewith, George T. & Aldridge, David (eds.)
1993 *Clinical Research Methodology for Complementary Therapies*, Hodder & Stoughton: London.

McKeown, Thomas
1976 *The Role of Medicine, Dream, Mirage or Nemesis*, Nuffield Provincial Hospitals Trust: London.

Pickstone, John V. (ed.)
1992 *Medical Innovations in Historical Perspective*, Macmillan: London.

Schmidt, Johannes G.
1994 "Measuring the Efficacy of Acupuncture", in: J.G. Schmidt & R.E. Steele (eds.): *Kritik der medizinischen Vernunft. Schritte zu einer zeitgemässen Praxis – Ein Lesebuch*, pp. 203-207, Mainz: Kirchheim.

Sich, Dorothea
1979 "*Naeng*. Begegnung mit einer Volkskrankheit in der modernen frauenärztlichen Sprechstunde in Korea", in: *Curare*, 2: 87-95.

Steffen, Vibeke
1995 Life Stories as Therapy – Autobiography and Myth in Alcoholics Anonymous, (unpublished).

Topley, Marjorie
1976 "Chinese Traditional Etiology and Methods of Care in Hong Kong", in: C. Leslie (ed.): *Asian Medical Systems: A Comparative Study*, pp. 243-265, University of California Press: Berkeley.

Young, Allan
1982 "The Anthropologies of Illness and Sickness", in: *Annual Review Anthropology*, 11: 257-85.

Bridging the Domains of Sound and Symptom in Tibetan and Allopathic Medicine: Cultural Phenomenology as Praxis

by Mary Ryan-Thorup

Recent research in psychoneuroimmunology shows that treatment with sound (music therapy) may result in a lessening of psychological and physical symptoms. This is one of the fundamental principles of Tibetan medicine. During eighteen months researching Tibetan medicine in Northern India, I observed over 1,000 patients being treated with a combination of herbal pills, diet and chanting of sacred Tibetan syllables. Based on observation and interviews, many showed marked improvement in health. These observations were on a case study basis, and led to a small randomized comparison study of the Tibetan treatment for osteo and rheumatoid arthritis, where patients showed significant improvements in limb movements with $P<0.0005$. How do Tibetan doctors explain the use of sound as an aid in the alleviation of sickness? The mind/body connection in Tibetan medicine is negotiated with the help of sacred sounds, or mantras. To understand Tibetan medical concepts of sound and their effects on the human body, a cultural phenomenology as praxis is suggested. The Tibetan Buddhist medical view linked with cultural phenomenology may help us articulate – in Western non-mechanistic terms – principles of sound and its healing effects.

Introduction

Over one and one-half years were spent in the Tibetan refugee community of Dharamsala, northern India (1991-1994). During this time, a randomized, controlled trial was undertaken comparing the Tibetan and local Western treatment for osteo and rheumatoid arthritis. It was found that the Tibetan medical treatment of herbal pills, diet, and spiritual practices resulted in lessening of arthritic symptoms with $P<0.0005$. During further clinical work, it became evident that the use of sound, of mantras, and of Tibetan Buddhist healing ceremonies based on chanting was an important part of most Tibetan treatments. In addition, it became clear that Tibetan Buddhist lama-practitioners and doctors understood effective principles underlying the use of sound in healing, or to alter the body's physiological functions. What can we learn from Tibetan medicine? Can we unravel their understanding of sound and its effects upon the body in a way conducive to dialogue between researchers of East and West?

Recently, in the field of cultural phenomenology in anthropology, a new understanding of the body has emerged which is referred to by various names: in terms of embodiment; being in the world; resonance and unification of subject and object. In these discussions, the boundaries of where the body begins and ends, and its connection to the mind, and exactly what constitutes "the Self" have been of primary interest. These themes reflect the philosophical nature of the debate, and how anthropologists are searching for a new framework for talking about the body/mind/self. As with most philosophy, and as with most theory, it is difficult to see how it plays out "on the ground", in the field, or as a workable repeatable event. Yet, in the realm of medicine and psychological healing, it is useful to have a frame of reference about mind/body interactions that prove of practical and significant help in treatment. Here, cultural phenomenological theories about the mind/body, and being in the world lack principles that can be applied in the healing of the mind/body. In this paper I hope to bring together different elements that could be called cultural phenomenology as praxis. This idea follows on the work of Professor Herbert Guenther (1994) in his use of hermeneutic phenomenology as a means for understanding ancient Tibetan Buddhist literature. We can extend his hermeneutics to encompass cultural phenomenology theory, thus developing a cultural phenomenology as praxis, taking it with us "in the field" so that we experience and understand indigenous knowledge in a way that is conducive to translation and research within a Western research tradition.

Within Tibetan Buddhist medicine and particularly their treatments for psychiatric disorders, there is a long tradition of the use of sound in the form of the chanting of sacred words, to alleviate both mind and body symptoms. Research by Herbert Benson at Harvard University proved that Tibetan Buddhist monks were able to radically alter their body chemistry with the use of sound and visualization. Also, in my fieldwork in northern India with a traditional Tibetan Buddhist doctor, I was able to document how the use of sound, with herbal pills and dietary restrictions, resulted in improved limb mobility and quality of life for arthritis patients. Thus, this paper is about how in Tibetan culture, certain scholars have developed the art of the use of sound to alleviate sickness, and alter the body's chemistry, and how they describe their system of the use of sound, and their anatomy of the "subtle body" that accounts for their success in this area. My main question is: how can we discern in other cultures their salient principles of healing – which have proven useful – so that they are applicable in the Western medical research context?

Previous Research on Tibetan Buddhist Uses of Sacred Sounds

According to some Tibetan doctors and Tibetan Buddhist lamas, the body can be controlled and manipulated using meditational techniques that rely on the use of sacred sounds, or mantras, and visualizations. These sounds and visualizations work to "pacify" the mind, and the pacification of the mind leads to physiological changes in the body.

Why should we consider the Tibetan understanding of the mind/body connection? What does Tibetan medicine, or Tibetan views of sound and healing, have to offer Western researchers?

One of the most thoroughly researched techniques of how meditation, with the use of sound and visualization, can be used to affect physiological functions was undertaken by Herbert Benson at Harvard. In 1979, Harvard cardiologist Herbert Benson received permission to study *gTummo*, or heat, the Tibetan meditation exercise in which experienced Tibetan Buddhist monks warm their near-naked bodies through meditation, even in freezing temperatures.

Herbert Benson documented the process of the monks conducting *gTummo*, while the monks wore soaking wet sheets. The room was approximately 5 degrees Celsius. At this temperature, the human body is programmed to shiver uncontrollably. Within five minutes, the monks, through chanting and visualization techniques, generated enough body heat that the sheets they wore began to steam, fogging the lenses of the research cameras. Within half an hour, the sheets were dry. The monks repeated this exercise twice to verify the process.

In another experiment, the monks meditated at 19,000 feet above sea level, in only their thin cotton robes, when the temperature was below -17.7 degrees Celsius, and it was snowing. Benson measured heart rate, blood pressure and temperature of the body on ten different spots, on the bodies of all the monks. They showed that they were able to maintain temperatures warm enough that they did not shiver, but could continue in a relaxed state, periodically chanting, combined with quiet periods of meditation, until the next morning, when the monks shook the snow off themselves, and walked down the mountain to their monastery.

In Western physiology, mammals are known to maintain their body temperature through either furs, or with humans, first by shivering, and then wearing extra clothing. Bodily reflexes such as shivering are considered automatic reactions to cold in order to produce extra heat. At the same time, blood vessels constrict so that less heat is lost through the skin, preserving warmth for the internal organs. The *gTummo* monks were shown to abort this autonomic process. They did not shiver, and their skins stayed warm. According to Tibetan doctors and lamas, the monks were able to generate interior heat through concentrating on visualizing and expanding an internal energy called *lung*, (which means wind or air) located near the solar plexus. In addition, they chanted certain mantras that linked with the internal heat, thus amplifying the effect of the visualization (Benson et al. 1979).

Based upon this research, it is possible that the Tibetan Buddhist understanding of the mind/body can offer Western medical researchers clues as to how sounds and states of mind, or visualizations, can work to alter physiological processes.

The question then, is not *what* Tibetan culture can offer Western sound therapy researchers, but *how:* How do Tibetan Buddhist healers and practitioners of Mantrayana, or "the path of sound," describe their understanding of sound, and the way it affects the human body? To answer this question, I turn to the basic tenets of Tibetan medicine, and the Tibetan medical view of the subtle body and channels.

Tibetan Medicine

The principles of Tibetan medicine are rooted in Vajrayana Buddhist philosophy. According to the oral tradition, along with knowledge of the religious teachings of the Buddhas, scholars brought with them the knowledge of healing taught by Sakyamuni Buddha 2000 years ago, and mixed it with the indigenous medical knowledge of the Bon shamans of Tibet.

To most Tibetan Buddhist healers and lamas, the ultimate cause of disease is that we are all living in what Tibetan Buddhism calls *samsara*, or illusion. Until we become enlightened, we will suffer from disease. Thus, enlightenment, or freedom from "obscuration" or "delusion", is the ultimate in health. Another way this is said by Tibetan Buddhist healers is, *"nothing exists independent of the mind"* (Ryan 1991:32). Buddhism differs from other religious systems in that the "Buddha," is not a god-like figure that is meant to be worshipped. Buddhism is more like a psychological manual, where the original practitioner became enlightened, free from all suffering, and able to heal others. Thus, practitioners of Buddhism turn to the writings of Gautauma Buddha, and other teachers after him who also became enlightened, in order to learn methods for discovering the nature of the mind, and the ultimate nature of reality. Another basic tenet of Buddhism is that one can depend on one's own experience and apprehension of the world to investigate the teachings of Buddhism, rather than following the Buddhist doctrines based on pure faith. The path is a personal investigation, and Buddhists say it leads to an understanding of oneself and reality, ultimately toward the end of being able to help others.

Within the context of their medical system, *"health is the result of harmony between the microcosm – the human mind/body vehicle – and the macrocosm – the universe. . . Disease is the result of disruption of this relationship by humans"* (Ryan 1991: 33). According to Dr. Dhadon, the human mind/body vehicle goes beyond its physical boundaries and encompasses a vast arena of invisible currents and vibratory structures, from both the inner mind of an individual, to cosmic and planetary forces acting upon this vehicle.

To discern the different levels of cause, the cause of disease in Tibetan medicine can be understood as both ultimate and proximate. The ultimate cause of all disease is ignorance, or unenlightenment and obscuration. If individuals were to understand the essence of their "true nature" as "perfection," as the "beautiful cosmic interplay of the universe in individual form," there would be no ignorance, and therefore, no bad actions, with the resulting bad karma and disease extending over many lifetimes. According to a Tibetan doctor and lama, Namkhai Norbu Rinpoche, it is the *sense* of separation from the "source" which is the cause of all illness (pc 1995). This separation is a separation of consciousness, as according to "cosmic law," humans could not incarnate without being part of the "one source" (pc 1995). Thus, it is the mind's thought of separation that creates this condition of separation and, consequently, the root of all ignorance, which leads to excessive emotions and, subsequently, disease. Another ultimate cause of disease is "karma," or *le*. It is defined by Dr. Dhadon as the organization of cosmic forces in reverberation to past actions, good or bad, and past afflictive emotions, or uncontrolled urges. These ideas of causality underline the importance of the mind and emotions in Tibetan medicine, and how it can influence the condition of the body and the surrounding environment.

Like Ayurvedic medicine, Tibetan medicine has a three-part division of humors. The three humors (*Nyes-Ba*) in Tibetan medicine are responsible for the normal mental and physical functions of an individual, and are one of the proximate causes of disease. When they are thrown out of balance, disease results. The three humors are: wind (*rLung*), bile (*mKhripa*) and phlegm (*bad-gan*). Other proximate causes of disease are called "conditions", such as season, diet, behavior and evil spirits.

Diagnosis is made by pulse, urine, interview and observation. The last part of diagnosis depends upon listening intently to the mind-set of the patient, so that spiritual and practical, emotional advice can be given. For example, a doctor may suggest that a patient see a certain lama for a specific ceremony that may end the patient being tormented by certain fears.

Treatment is based primarily on herbal preparations, the use of mantras, or sacred syllables, and diet and personal advice. As the focus of this paper is on the use of sound, or mantras or chanting in Tibetan Buddhist medicine, I shall focus on the subtle anatomy charts in Tibetan medicine, and the way they understand how sounds are registered in the body, affecting physiological changes.

The Subtle Body and Channels in Tibetan Physiology

The subtle channels
Within the subtle body, there are said to be numerous psychic channels (*rtsa*), airs or forces (*rlung*), and essences (*thig-le*). These three are the main components of the subtle body, and they provide the link between the gross physical body and what is called the "vajra" or diamond body, the spiritual body.

The psychic nerves or channels are numerous; they are sometimes numbered 72,000. There are three main channels: the central vein (*dbu-ma*); the right channel (*ro-ma*); and the left channel (*rkyang-ma*).

The central channel runs from the top of the head beneath the soft spot on the skull, to a space located four finger-widths beneath the navel. The channel represents the absolute aspect, consciousness, non-dual wisdom. The vein is straight, hollow, luminous and blue. It is said to be as thin as an arrow shaft. It is not the same as the spinal cord, but corresponds to it. It is the subtle vertical axis of the subtle body, as the spine is the gross one.

The right column branches off from the central one just above the eyebrows and runs parallel to the central one, an inch or so away from it, rejoining it just above the lowest part of it just below the navel. The left column follows the same path on that side of the body. This is the way it is visualized in meditation, yet in practice, the two sides intertwine with the central channel at various points.

Both side veins are thinner than the central channel, and are described as hollow and luminous. The right vein is said to be red and represents the feminine aspect, blood, and most importantly, the basic desire-grasping obscuration.

The left side is white. It represents the male aspect, the element water and the basic hatred-aversion obscuration. When the airs and essences in the three veins are consciously held together where the three join the navel, with the proper mantras, the mystic heat (*gTummo*) arises.

The subtle airs contain the life-force or *sRog-rLung*. The Tibetan doctors and lamas view a reciprocal character between mind and the life-air, so that controlling and stabilizing the airs also stabilize the mind. This relationship can be understood when we think how our breathing pattern alters depending upon our mental and emotional state. We have only to think of the difference in breathing when we are feeling angry, or concentrating. Thus, the mind is affected through the use of the breath, and through the use of sound.

The chakras
In Tibetan medicine and Tantric Buddhist practices, different chakra systems are used. In general, there are six major chakras. The chakras, or psychic centers (*khor-lo*), are the circular centers formed on the central column by the intersection of many subtle veins and the collection of various essences. It is said that when the chakras are purified and fully opened, they become the internal mandalas of the Five Innate Buddhas.

The number of veins at each chakra accounts for the number of "petals" or spokes of the wheel associated with each. The colors, sounds and elements associated with each chakra reflect the specific aspects of consciousness which the chakra represents. Within each chakra is contained a particular sound, that when uttered or sung, results in the harmonization of that area of the body.

The use of mantras
Mantras, or sacred sounds, which may be a deity's name, a concept or spiritual "realm," are considered words of power, which through proper usage, can pacify and clear the mind. Mantras are thought of as primordial syllables that have healing properties both for self-healing, and healing others.

According to one of the medical tantras used by Dr. Lady Dhadon, the subtle body is the energy body, and energy is manifest as vibration. In the impure, unrealized, diseased body, the vibrational sounds are discordant and unclear. According to Dr. Dhadon, by practising the recitation of mantras, one can readjust the vibrational harmony of the subtle body and realize it as the Buddha-body. Mantras are not repeated like a parrot, but may contain a sacred idea or visualization, or may be said in a state of repose and introspection. It is considered to be a tool for thinking in Tibetan culture. It is said that by calling forth a particular sound, one calls forth its content into a state of immediate reality. Tibetans say that words and their sounds are like deeds. Often a Tibetan lama will say, *"Be careful what you wish for!"*, as thinking can result in materialization. In Tibetan medicine different mantras are used, depending upon the ailment, by both the practitioner and the patient. I have witnessed many cases of warts, epilepsy and other conditions being curtailed by mantras, and also witnessed in my own research on arthritis how the use of mantras acted to pacify and clear the patient's mind, perhaps acting as an impetus for the healing effect of the herbal pills also used.

It is said that mantras are also used to "tune in" to the basic inherent Buddha nature within the patient. Mantras are particularly used in the case of mental disorders, since they are said to readjust the consciousness of the patient.

Special forms of healing rely on the correspondence between certain mantras and subtle channels and veins. In one healing process, the subtle veins and channels are said to have specific crossing points, where specific mantric syllables "live," the saying of which can heal these points instantaneously. If these points are blocked, it is said that the vibration has been blocked, and the flesh in these areas can be hardened as a result. The mantric sounds are said to exist in the psychic veins blended with the airs.

The use of sound in the form of sacred mantras pervades all aspects of Tibetan life. Every moment of every day is filled with the recitation of mantras: over the rising of the sun in the morning; the collection of water and firewood; during walks; preparing food etc. Herbert Benson's research points to the necessity of considering further how Tibetans have made advances in their understanding of the mind/body connection, and the use of sound to alter states of consciousness and bodily processes. Mantric prayers in Tibetan can be understood as combining the powerful effects of poetry, which create images that relax the mind beyond logical thought, and music, which enters the human into a more subtle interaction and expression of the inner life.

Cultural Phenomenology as Praxis: Linking with Tibetan Buddhist Medicine

Within anthropology, there are a number of researchers who have used the theoretical orientations of phenomenology to understand their field experiences with indigenous medical practitioners and healers. For example, Thomas Csordas (1994), Rene Devisch (1993), Carol Lederman (1991) and Robert Dejarlais (1992) have all written about the relationship between aesthetics and healing. While all of these researchers contribute descriptions of aesthetic encounters of sound, color and symbols that affect psychobiological changes, none of them offer an actual theory of how aesthetics can affect self-awareness, and how this change in self-awareness results in changes in states of illness and disease on both a local and social level. Rather, they use the theoretical orientations of phenomenology descriptively, giving anecdotal evidence of the efficacy of indigenous healing events, both on a macro- and microsocial level. None are able to explain what *mediates* a change in psychobiological symptoms as a result of aesthetic encounters of sound, color and symbols.

In Herbert Guenther's work with Tibetan Buddhist texts, he uses the method of hermeneutical phenomenology to *"open up to the multi-levels of experience"* that are latent in the Tibetan texts themselves (1991: 13). According to Guenther and others (Levin 1991), phenomenology is a process of disclosure, of revelation, of epiphany. In the context of discourse, it can be thought of as truth as constant, attentive disclosure, versus the more static truth of correctness (Levin

1991). In this way, Guenther opens himself to the Tibetan texts as poetry, in which he participates in a relationship that extends beyond the boundaries of his known world of understanding.

By engaging in a cultural phenomenology as praxis, we can apply the basic tenets of hermeneutical phenomenology to understanding Tibetan medicine on its many different levels, opening-up to the "Other" and their understanding of the way sound can initiate a healing event both physically and psychologically. Cultural phenomenology offers a methodology for going beyond our own cultural limitations to understanding other people's ways of understanding health and the use of sound to heal. It requires that researchers become involved with indigenous medical practitioners in the playing-out of their healing rituals and practices on a day-to-day basis in their own context, and then allowing this experience and knowledge to be hermeneutically translated back into the western research paradigms.

As mentioned in the previous section, in Tibetan Buddhist medicine, the use of chanting, of visualization and of sacred healing texts read aloud – basically the use of aesthetics – carry experiential meaning; they refer to levels of meaning of which most Tibetans (and now myself) are aware. The texts and healing ceremonies refer to the subtle anatomy of the body as a reality that can be altered, that can affect physiological change. According to Dr. Dhadon, the metaphors in the healing chants and texts *are true to the extent that we open to them*, making them true within our own being. In contrast to truths recognized in positivism, these truths are truthful only to the extent that they succeed in soliciting our reflective awareness and bring about a transformation – first in our consciousness, followed by our body and our relationships – of our experience.

Through cultural phenomenology as praxis, we are able to understand the Tibetan medical explanation for sound as a tool for healing. This paper only tentatively addresses the way we can open to Tibetan medical frameworks of the use of sound in healing. Yet it is hoped that by beginning with a description of the subtle body anatomy used in Tibetan medicine, and mantric healing, we may begin to approach Tibetan ways of seeing that result in a respective dialogue between Eastern and Western ways of using sound in healing. The Western, process-oriented, open-ended framework of a hermeneutic cultural phenomenology makes it possible for us to understand these ancient Tibetan teachings and to reach beyond our ethnocentric mode of enquiry into cross-cultural models of health and healing.

References

Clifford, Terry
1984   *Tibetan Buddhist Medicine and Psychiatry: The Diamond Healing*, York Beach Maine: Samuel Weiser.

Csordas, Thomas
1980   *The Sacred Self: A Cultural Phenomenology of Charismatic Healing*, University of California Press: Berkeley.

Dejarlais, Robert
1992   *Body and Emotion: The Aesthetics of Illnes and Healing in the Nepal Himalayas*, University of Pennsylvania Press: Philadelphia.

Devisch, Rene
1993   *Weaving the Threads of Life: The Khita Gyn-Eco-Logical Healing Cult among the Yaka*, University of Chicago Press: Chicago.

Guenther, Herbert
1994   *Wholeness Lost and Wholeness Regained: Forgotten Tales of Individuation from Ancient Tibet*, SUNY Series in Buddhist Studies, State University of New York Press: New York.

Merleau-Ponty, Maurice
1962   *Phenomenology of Perception*, Northwestern University Press: Evanston, Ill.

Ryan, Mary
1994   "Measuring the Efficacy of an Indigenous Remedy: The Tibetan Medical Treatment for Rheumatoid and Osteoarthritis", publication pending, Social Science and Medicine, rights preliminarily reserved, from author by request.

The Development of Music Therapy Research as a Perspective of Complementary Medicine

by David Aldridge

Complementary medical approaches in Europe have seen a demand for research initiatives over the past ten years. Music therapy, as such an approach, has faced this challenge too and in this paper I will present how some of the problems have been recognised and resolved. A number of individual researchers, based in different countries, have attempted to promote music therapy research.

Music therapy, like nursing, psychotherapy and various other forms of helping professions, is being challenged to produce research results. The source of that challenge is coming both from within the profession itself, and from without. From within the profession, a new generation of music therapists is demanding academic credibility, and this need is linked to the establishment of postgraduate music therapy courses leading to masters qualifications. Music therapists, too, are demanding within their own career trajectories that they can deepen their understanding of what they are doing and gain academic credentials by further study. Combined with this internal demand, we are seeing throughout the European Union a demand for outcomes research related to varying therapeutic initiatives both from third-party funders and from employing health institutions. With government cutbacks in health and education, enhanced scrutiny in university spending, and fiscal demands for efficiency and productivity, then music therapy departments are having to either justify their existence by producing material evidence of their efficacy or produce research papers to improve their academic points rating.

This means that a relatively new profession is being forced to develop research results without having had the chance to establish research training, without a satisfactory background of research material and without the opportunity to negotiate an acceptable way of doing research that is related to therapeutic outcome. Indeed, we are not alone in this; rehabilitation medicine and general medical practice in the Western world stand under the same spotlight of scrutiny.

In addition, we are faced with a relative lack of research expertise. Some of us have a research career that has experience of various forms of research projects. However, few of our colleagues have had the opportunity to do postgraduate research and are being expected to teach research methods and supervise research projects. While this may be a necessity, driven by need, I suggest that in some cases we will find that colleagues are being prepared for an over-idealised world of academic research, that reflects maybe the lack of experience within the profession, rather than research that is focused upon clinical practice. It is vital that we develop a sound basis of research-orientated clinical practitioners.

However, within Europe there are several moves that have been underway during the last ten years to provide a research infrastructure within individual countries, and which I hope will meet the challenge to cooperate on an international basis. Many of us are trying to provide research support that suits the complementary therapists themselves, while serving their needs to reach out to a wider community of professional colleagues.

Research Purposes

At the heart of much of this debate is the difference between process research and outcomes research. Many creative arts therapists, for instance, will be interested in what happens when they perform their art as therapy. Music therapists ask the question, how does the music unfold and what has this to do with the changing status of the person with whom I am working? This changing status may be musical, aesthetic, psychological, clinical or indeed social. External parties, however, may be more concerned with the differences before a person has music therapy when compared with what happens after a person has had music therapy. The question will be related to the material benefit associated with doing music therapy. This question is not so much concerned with how that process is carried out; rather, it is concerned with the actual clinical outcome itself (and sometimes the costs incurred related to that outcome). Within the whole field of health care delivery in the Western world, such questions are being placed in the foreground of research initiatives.

Table 1: Purposes of research

masters and doctoral theses	inward-looking	individual focus, often process based
doctoral project as part of institutional research program	linked to an established, project can be broader	individual and group; process or outcomes
project specific	outward-looking	group needs; tends towards outcomes research

Furthermore, there is also a difference between the purposes of research. At the moment, in the junior profession of music therapy we have researchers preparing masters material and doctoral studies. These studies are often of a different nature to postgraduate research studies and research contracted to outside agencies. Doctoral studies are focused on the development of the doctoral candidate. They are there for the sole process of developing someone who will later be able to carry out research. Therefore, the work itself will often be of an intensely deep and inward-looking nature. The research that is carried out by experienced researchers will be more outward looking and often be at the request of some external agency wanting to see some material benefit from their investment. Therefore, the purposes and the methods used will differ. I am arguing that we need both these forms of research, and only to foster an inward-looking research will restrict the nature of music therapy research, and thereby practice, in the future. As a rational step forward, single case research designs are a positive way forward fostering both process-oriented work combined with the possibility for assessing outcomes.

Science as Performed Knowledge

What kind of research we do, and the methods we use to go about researching, will be influenced by the philosophy of science that we have. My main proposal is that science is a process, an activity and not a set of commandments set in stone for all time as the basis for a dogma. In a postmodern world, where all the major themes are challenged and deconstructed, then it is our responsibility to construct themes that are appropriate to the knowledge that we need. While this debate is often set out as differences in truth claims, that is, "Is truth relative?" or "Is there one truth?", my argument is that such a position belongs to a previous era of debate. Claims about truth have already been discussed in various other scientific disciplines. What we are really making claims about are objectivity and subjectivity. And this debate can be currently found in the nursing literature, in the world of psychology, in journals dedicated to social science and particularly over the last ten years in the field of complementary medicine.

First, let me make an observation about science in a broad sense. The word science itself in its English usage springs from the Latin *scire*, to know, originally meaning to cut, and thereby to decide, and has a relationship with the Latin adjective *scius*, that means "knowing". So, on the one hand we have a derivation of science that appears to be about making decisions, to cut and to separate. Or, we can follow another route and look at the adjective *scius* as it refers to knowing, and as it occurs in the Latin word *conscius*, literally con=together, scius=knowing). Perhaps this is what we are searching for in our scientific activity; how we can share knowledge, or how can we bring knowledge into consciousness.

Yet another perspective would take us to the German word for science, *wissenschaft*. *Wissen* is to know or to know about, and is related to knowledge and judgement, and *schaffen* is to make or create, or to manage or accomplish. So, from another European perspective we can see science as the activity of creating knowledge, and perhaps it is this creative activity that may appeal to many of us today, and perhaps some of us feel has become lost to the scientific activity. Knowledge is something that can be done; it is a creative activity, a process, not a fixed product. Indeed the word knowledge in English is distantly derived from a root that means "I can" (Middle English: *Ic can*, German: *können* and *kennen*) and is perhaps best described as the statement "I can know". Once we take such a position of knowledge being actively acquired, then we can speculate upon the various arts of doing science.

This is a move away from the Cartesian position that separates mind and body as reflected in *cogito ergo sum* – I think therefore I am. What I am proposing here is *ago ergo sum* – I perform therefore I am.

What remains to be added to these descriptions from the Latin and the German roots is the notion of decision or judgement; therefore, doing science – or the activity of sciencing – is a matter of deciding. It is therefore a moral activity.

How do we create knowledge, then? This question lies at the centre of many modern scientific debates, and is a question of methodology. One of our critiques of modern science doing is that the argument rarely concentrates on the subject matter of our inquiry that leads to a new creative discovery for the person who wants to know. The activity of science seems more like the pressure for us to conform in our knowing to a set of prescriptions that are applied to a given body of knowledge, that is, methodolatry not methodology. It is this struggle with an appropriate methodology that we find in the current creative arts therapy literature, and one that has been hotly debated during the last decade within other fields of applied therapeutic practice .

We see this breaking out in the debate about quantitative or qualitative research, where one is proposed as the only form of research inquiry. While music therapists in the United States, partly because of their education structure, have a tradition of music therapy research, that tradition has often been polarised into two opposing camps: qualitative research versus quantitative research. The grounds for this polarisation appear to be historically-based in the establishment of a political professional identity within the field of practice. What some of us have been trying to do is to avoid such polarisation and foster a climate of tolerance that allows us to develop music therapy research that suits music therapists and their various purposes. All too often this debate has been at the foreground of research initiatives and has masked the underlying political debate about which group should hold political sway within the profession. We could just as easily translate this debate into the intolerance of varying music therapy schools for one another. Such arguments really are superfluous at a time when the profession itself is ripe to develop, and in its maturity should be ready to extend the tolerance necessary for knowing together.

What I am arguing for is that if science is a creative doing of knowledge, then the way that we can do knowledge about being human is not restricted to instrumentation through machines; rather, knowledge is something that can be sung, or played, or danced or acted. Underlying this approach is a philosophy of the world that moves away from a solely materialistic perspective to a perspective that sees the world as a living organism improvised in the moment in which we are all taking part.

If truth in postmodern society is relative, and the self is constructed to meet the variety of life's contingencies, then we move away from the model of one generation initiating the next generation into the truths of its own beliefs. Instead, we have a pool of experts and advisers to whom we can turn for advice. In some modern alternative healing approaches, traditional forms of teaching by initiation and learning by apprenticeship, are rejected in favour of an eclecticism that takes techniques assembled according to the situation. A new generation of music therapists is being trained that demands a choice of learning approaches which suits their approach to music and to therapy. The pioneer approach of the teacher/pupil relationship no longer holds sway, and while the restriction of the relationship may be lost, so too is the security. Furthermore, as there is no established tradition of music therapy research, we have the luxury of deciding what methods are appropriate to use in our scientific endeavour. While some of us will research alone, others will decide to work together in groups. What we need to avoid is that one group can make an exclusive claim to determine the doing of knowledge according to their own principles. To establish tolerance we need to understand each other and our varying purposes.

The activity of doing research, or sciencing as knowing, is concerned not with restricting us to a one-dimensional sense of being according to an accepted orthodox world view, but the possibility for the interpretation of the self as new. What we choose to know, and how we know is a matter of judgement, and therefore one of moral agency. How each one of us decides to know in the future, with whom we share that knowledge, and how we tolerate and incorporate what others know, will determine the scientific culture of music therapy.

Research Ideas in Practice

We see from the differing phases in Table 2 that there are continuing themes related to our work. These themes are related to the needs of our colleagues in practice. The theme of physiological change was chosen because it met the needs of colleagues with whom we were working, and within the University we were closely integrated with the Department of Physiology. The clinical research continues and forms the backbone of our published material as the main area of interest for clinicians is clinical practice. What I hope to do with this clinical work, however, is to graft that work onto the underlying theoretical structures that exist within our music therapy approach and within clinical practice in general. This is surely the purpose of an academic department. Such clinical and theoretical work then leads outwards into the world with various publications and inwards by feeding the teaching of the music therapy students in training.

Table 2: Four research themes continuing over three working phases

	Physiological work	Clinical applications	Theoretical work	Publication
Phase One	establish physiological criteria of change in therapist/patient interaction	single case studies, develop working methods appropriate to a therapy setting	literature reviews, theory development	case studies and position papers
Phase Two	refine hypotheses and test out methods, establish experimental method	develop working relationships with the hospital staff, attempt feasibility study of cooperative work	collect case examples from recorded work	case studies and clinical outcome material
Phase Three	continue work, identify clinical problems and refine hypotheses	look for larger scale clinical trials, establish contacts with other clinical groups	develop theory and refine techniques	develop database produce collected works CD ROM

Publication plays an important role in that it encourages therapists to reflect upon their practice and to move from an idiosyncratic language to a common language suitable for a variety of clinical practitioners. I am not advocating that creative arts therapists abdicate their own language, rather that they negotiate a common language with others to form a community of practitioners. What has emerged both in the field of creative arts therapies and in other forms of complementary medicine is that we have practitioners who have not been trained to write for academic journals. Part of our responsibility as academic researchers and editors is not simply to decry a lack of standards but bring into being the possibility for practitioners to learn to write.

Research Training

Coupled to the need for research training and an expectation of written material we have tried to introduce an element of research teaching in the second year of the masters training program through individually-based, case-oriented research or small-scale research projects.

While it is possible to gain a doctoral qualification (*doctor rerum medizinum*: allied to medicine) within the faculty of medicine at the University of Witten Herdecke, we have also seen the necessity that the Danish University of Aalborg doctoral program identified, and that is for the establishment of a specific qualification of Doctor of Music Therapy. When music therapists want to gain a higher qualification, they want it to be related directly to their own discipline, thus the naming of the qualification is bound to the status requirements of the profession and its recognition within an academic culture.

It has been necessary for our institute to cooperate with others. When we have a limited, albeit valuable, experience and expertise, it makes sense then to pool that expertise and knowledge between university centres. It is only by our differing countries coming together that we can begin to meet the research challenges that are being made of us. Within our program we have initiated a literature support service that is being shared currently with Denmark, Holland and the other Nordic countries. This database has been based on our recognition of the need for a simple research support service within Germany to meet the needs of students who have trained with us and are now colleagues in practice. In addition, there are other colleagues who do not have the benefit of institutional support and it is our responsibility to at least support them in whatever way we can, should they wish to begin clinical research. All too often the best resources are directed to universities and other less fortunate colleagues are left without adequate support. It seems unfair to accuse them of not developing research initiatives if we do not provide them with a research infrastructure to pursue the questioning of their clinical practice. This has meant that we do not expect that every contact for research advice will come to fruition as a doctoral study, rather that we can encourage questioning and disciplined thinking through everyday practice that will have a timing and agenda according to the needs and capacities of the practitioners.

In addition, we also see the need to offer research methodological advice, and in some cases specific teaching. I see no reason why this should be restricted to our own national interests and call upon my colleagues to find a way in which we can collaborate to offer a European "college," in the sense of a group that will offer such support. Such an aim is surely the basis of European funding.

Conclusion

It is important that we continue to further establish European connections. One way to accomplish this will be by exchanging teaching staff interested in research, or providing the opportunity for extended visits. Promoting research placements for higher-level students, or junior members of staff, is also a possibility that can benefit institutions. For example, we have had visiting music therapists who have sat in on the teaching sessions, experienced a series of therapy sessions and made a review of literature on a theme that has interested them. There are a number of institutions throughout Europe that have special areas of interest for music therapists, and an extended working visit is a good way of getting to know other institutions. A significant step would be for junior practitioners to work in other settings and thereby gain new experiences. While some clinical practitioners may not wish to work in an academic environment forever, giving them a chance to work for a short period of time with colleagues in academia brings new understandings for all concerned. In the long term, relationships are made that foster research opportunities in clinical practice.

We certainly need to collaborate on providing a research infrastructure. By this I mean that we have to share our various resources for offering methodological advice and teaching research methods. There is enough expertise, even if scattered throughout several centres. The problem remains of how to utilise and coordinate such expertise. We have access to databases and literature archives within our institute. What we do not have, as yet, is a means of giving a broad access to such material, although with the advent of CD Rom technology it is possible to share a large amount of data both as text databases and as video and musical material. What we do need are cooperating centres within the different countries, but that would mean that institutes would also have to communicate and cooperate with each other rather than simply exchange intentions. In terms of teaching expertise, we could all benefit from collaborating our various expertise. In the field of therapist supervision and research supervision there are scant resources available as to how we teach such supervision, yet there is surely a common pool of experience that could be explicated into practical guidelines or a working paper.

One important way forward would be to promote a "single-case" agency where we could coordinate single case methods teaching, offer suitable research formats and collect research examples. By doing this we could develop a set of clinical studies as a clinical studies database. This would necessitate translating the clinical studies into a common set of European languages, but would offer clinical researchers a pool of comparative data.

References

Aldridge, David
1990   "The development of a research strategy for music therapists in a hospital setting", in: *The Arts in Psychotherapy*, 17: 231-237.

1991   "Aesthetics and the individual in the practice of medical research: a discussion paper", in: *Journal of the Royal Society*, 84: 147-150.

1992   "The needs of individual patients in clinical research", in: *Advances*, 8: 58-65.

1993a   "Music therapy research: I. A review of the medical research literature within a general context of music therapy research. Special Issue: Research in the creative arts therapies", in: *Arts in Psychotherapy*, 20: 11-35.

1993b   "Music Therapy research: II. Research methods suitable for music therapy", in: *The Arts in Psychotherapy*, 20: 117-131.

1993c   "Single case research designs", in: G. Lewith and D. Aldridge (eds.): *Clinical Research Methodology for Complementary Therapies*, pp. 136-168, Hodder and Stoughton: London.

Aldridge, David, Brandt, Gudrun & Wohler, Dagmar
1989   "Towards a common language among the creative art therapies", in: *The Arts in Psychotherapy*, 17: 189-195.

Communicating Bodies

– when the cell goes cultural and the doctor goes bananas

by Helle Johannessen

Once I went for a sitting with a famous British clairvoyant called Ivor James. I had previously seen Ivor James perform in public, drawing pictures of persons identified as deceased relatives or friends of the audience, and forwarding messages from the dead to the living. I found his art quite fascinating, but had no particular wish to contact any dead kin. Urged by two friends – independently – I did, however, sign up for a sitting, thinking that perhaps there was some kind of "meaning" to this.

The sitting turned out to be quite an interesting session. Not one message was delivered from the dead to me. In fact, this was of no concern. Rather, we talked about the work of Ivor James, and about how he himself and most of his clients explained what happened during shows and sittings.

It so happened that I was acquainted with many of Ivor James' Danish clients. During my field work in the alternative sector of the Danish health care system, I worked in a New Age center where he was quite popular among staff and friends of the house. I had accompanied several persons immediately before and after sittings, and observed some being addressed during public shows. All of these clients firmly believed the drawings by James and the messages he spoke to be true revelations from "the other side," from the dead. They believed that Ivor James was able to actually "see" the spirits of the dead in the room and make a drawing of this "presence". Likewise, they believed that he could "hear" the voices of the spirits and thus convey messages and concerns.

During my conversation with Ivor James, it did, however, become clear to me, that he himself did not share this understanding of his abilities. He claimed neither to see any spirits of dead persons in the room nor hear any voices from spirits of another world. Instead, he explained that he was sensitive to the person(s) in front of him and the mental images evoked in this person. He was – at best – able to somehow tune into the mental dimension of his client and draw a picture created (unconsciously) by the client. He also pointed to the importance of the very tolerable attitude toward the pictures on behalf of the clients as an explanation of his "success". Most clients were hoping for contact with some deceased relative, and were more than willing to accept even the slightest resemblance of picture and person as proof of the true origin in the spirit of a beloved friend or relative.

James told me that he tried to tell his clients how he himself experienced the sessions, but soon discovered that it was not a good idea. Most did not understand him and, therefore, did not believe him. Those that did, stopped seeing him, probably because they did not want to get in touch with themselves, but with their deceased ones. To me – as an academic studying alternative medicine – the explanation offered by James did, however, seem much more plausible and interesting than the ones offered by his clients. I got quite excited.

To me, the session reflected the enormous flexibility in explanatory models for the same phenomena. James and his clients are engaged in the very same happenings, a sitting or a public show with drawings and spoken words shared openly, and yet they comprehend these as very distinct "events". They do not apply the same meaning to the happenings but interpret and explain the phenomena within two different cosmologies. Rather than querying into the question of which explanation is the true one, I find the interesting point to be that both are meaningful – but for two different audiences: the clients and the professionals.

This argument leads to a more general consideration of explanatory models in alternative therapy, their potentials and implications in different contexts. Is a general foundation of alternative theories in popular cosmology a main obstacle to communication between alternative therapists and conventional medical doctors as well as researchers with a critical approach? Common "sayings" (assumptions?) within alternative therapy may be very meaningful for Mrs. Jones looking up a therapist or the doctor/therapist making up his personal explanatory system. Both are using popular cosmologies of the contemporary West as their frame of reference. For sceptical conventional doctors and researchers, trained to be critical and look beyond the obvious and apparent, these explanatory models may, on the contrary, block meaningful understanding.

Could we start anew, and try to interpret the observed phenomena within scientific and scholarly frames of reference? That quest is the main focus of my paper. By applying newer scientific models and theories representing somewhat the same pattern or organizational logic as the popular models, I suggest some explanations of the very same phenomena, potentially more acceptable for academics.

When the Cell Goes Cultural

From a scholarly perspective, one major problem with popular explanatory models for alternative therapy is that metaphors and concepts often point to a very anthropomorphic image of the world, a world where anything from molecules to galaxies is imbued with human abilities such as to think and choose. A fascinating idea. The problem is just that this idea inevitably leads to the question: *who* is thinking and choosing? I? My T-lymphocytes? All of them? My knees? The Earth? The Moon? The Milky Way? All of it? What a cacophony of thinking and choosing. And what a world, thoroughly inhabited by homunculi at every possible level of abstraction. Similarly, it is a world where invisible features become human-like spirits – be they spirits of deceased or (super)natural forces; and anything not readily explanatory within common sense is referred to as something "spiritual" or "energetic".

On behalf of these general images or assumptions, the world seems quite densely populated with humanized, conscious, spiritual beings of energy, all trying to manipulate or direct the "real" humans to a more human way of living. The image seems like one of mirrors in mirrors, where all man can see is himself in a variety of sizes, shapes and significance in a giant human-like hologram.

No matter how fascinating this view seems, the implicated homunculi at all levels represent a logical problem bound to create offence in academic circles. Paradoxically, exactly this characteristic which turns academics off seems to be attractive to clients. A world represented in the image of man makes you feel safely at home because it resembles your daily life-experiences. The "invisible" – be it cells and molecules hidden in the interior of the body, dead persons or natural forces – is conceptualized in models well founded in popular cosmology. The cell goes cultural in the sense that humans anthropomorphize anything from molecules to galaxies and envision that anything is able to think and choose.

Communicating Bodies

In suggesting other explanations for the phenomena experienced in alternative therapy, I draw heavily on the semiotic approach founded by Charles Sanders Peirce at the end of the last century. Fundamental in semiotics is a conceptual and analytical split between (1) a sign, (2) the object referred to by the sign, and (3) the interpreter linking the sign and the object. This is most often illustrated by this model:

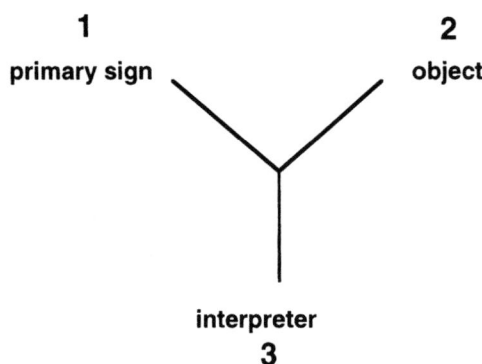

Figure 1

Without delving into details of semiotics, I will stress a main assumption behind this model: that man does not see the "object" in itself freed from subjective bias. Rather, this is considered impossible. Whatever sensed is considered a "sign" that is interpreted by somebody, and only in this process the "object" appears. Basically, it is a model implying communication as a main characteristic of all happenings. We do not really "see" or "hear" the world as it is. We (interpreters) communicate with selected "significant" appearances (signs) in the world, and in this communication, we construct local images of the world (objects). Perhaps it is worthwhile to stress that the term "object" is used in a quite abstract and general way. It does not necessarily refer to a "thing", but may as well refer to an event, a narrative, or something else. In this context, the object simply represents the actual conceptualization of whatever sign is observed. Any object is produced by an interpreter's linking of signs to specific concepts, things, or happenings which are meaningful in the cosmology of the interpreter. The object, thus, must correspond to some properties of the sign, as well as to properties of the interpreter's general cosmology.

One of the qualities of this model is that it can be expanded to include several interpreters and objects referring to the same sign. Two persons can view the same sign and produce very different objects of this. This was what happened with Ivor James and his clients. They participated in the same happening, but objectified it differently. In the semiotic model, this can be illustrated as in figure 2.

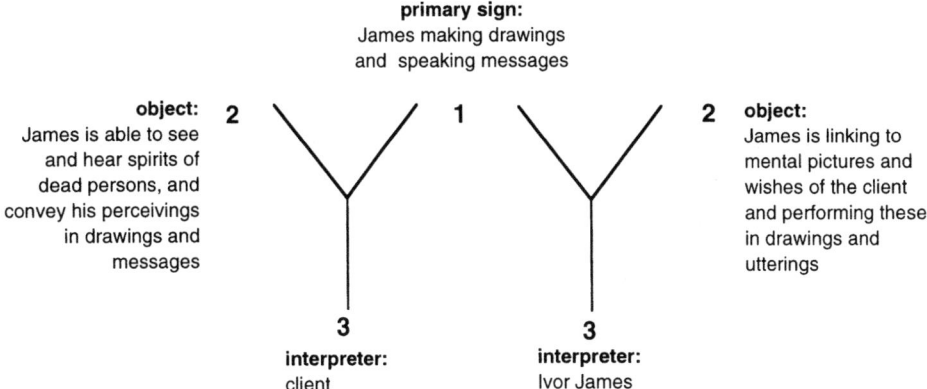

Figure 2

The interpreter's linking of sign and object is based on qualitative likeness. That means that some qualitative correspondence between the sign and the object is recognized by the interpreter and forms the rationale of the link established. The likeness or correspondence is not of "kind". One is a sign and the other an object; they belong to different logical levels. The correspondence is, rather, one of structural resemblance in that similar, fundamental qualitative patterns are refound in both sign and object and form the rationale for the link. In the example of James and his clients, the clients recognized structural likeness between the faces drawn by James and some deceased friends or relatives and, thus, interpreted and objectified the drawings as portraits of these deceased persons. James, on the other hand, knew that he did not see any spirits and, therefore, interpreted his apparent success with the portraits as a sign that he was able to link to mental pictures of his clients.

In view of the semiotic model and the basic assumptions behind it, it may be fruitful to look for structural patterns implicated by the general anthropomorphic image, presented above, and then look for scientific models with corresponding qualitative patterns.

What is the general structural pattern implied in the common assumption that at all levels of the universe, from molecules to galaxies, one finds intelligence and entities able to think and choose? I suggest that one basic principle of the pattern is "difference," recognized differences in the course of diseases and healing, i.e., or in biological processes in general. In noting the *variety* in the course of similar phenomena as a significant sign, the emphasis is on an apparent non-mechanical structure of biological processes in the body, in nature, in cosmos. In searching for models of a non-mechanical kind, the most experience-near model is found in man himself; and in the search for basic models of non-mechanical processes, intelligence, thinking and choosing are apt candidates in a popular cosmology. The cells, the molecules, the organs and the body at large are imbued with intelligence in order to explain non-mechanical processes leading to variety and diversity in biology.

That biological processes can be non-mechanical is not – I believe – conflicting academic cosmology of today. The time when Nature was likened to a clock work is long gone. Thus, the fundamental structural characteristic behind the alternative model should not pose a problem in itself. We just have to objectify it in different terms and within a different frame of reference.

Rather than talking of intelligence as a universal principle, I suggest that we talk about *semiosis* as a universal principle. In this, I follow the Danish biochemist, Jesper Hoffmeyer, who has introduced the concept of a "semiosphere" interpenetrating all other "spheres", such as the biosphere, atmosphere, hydrosphere, etc. According to Hoffmeyer, the semiosphere consists of communication in the widest sense: *"sounds, fragrants, movements, colours, forms, electrical fields, heat radiation, waves of many kinds, chemical signals, touch etc. In short, signs of life"* (Hoffmeyer 1994: 7) (my translation).

By introducing the semiosphere Hoffmeyer wants to supplement the dominating ecological understanding, which he claims to be stuck at a physical-chemical level. We tend to neglect that all organisms, plants and animals are primarily living in a world of "significance and meaning". *"Anything sensed by an organism means something to it: food, escape, propagation – or despair, for that matter. For man lives in the biosphere as well"* (ibid: 8) (my translation).

In Hoffmeyer's model, significance and meaning at all levels are realized by relegating the essence of the semiotic process to local entities at tissue or cell level. Tissues and cells are able to interpret their environment and act upon this interpretation. In this model, the body is not a collection of mechanics governed by the brain. Nor is the brain function, as we normally think of it (intelligence, thinking), distributed in the body. The body is an organism comprised of billions of smaller organisms all engaged in the biosemiotic process. All are interacting with their local environment, being exposed to an enormous amount of stimuli, but only reacting to a few selected ones in a way based on the relation between the organism and stimuli in question. Rather than imagining the body as a hierarchical entity with hierarchies of communication (like brain-governs-body, or DNA-governs-embryology) Hoffmeyer suggests it should be conceptualized as a self-organizing chaos. To illustrate what is meant by this, he refers to a bee swarm where thousands of bees are able to coordinate their activities of collecting nectar, breeding larvas etc., without any central government. This is managed by the thousands of local activities of communication (signs and interpretations) continually going on (Hoffmeyer 1994: 134-6). Variation is not based in thinking and choosing, but in local communication and very often new variations occur through misinterpretation of (otherwise well-known) stimuli with new patterns as a consequence.

In Hoffmeyer's work, I see some very positive qualities. One is his persistence on the importance of communication, meaning and significance for processes at all levels of the biosphere; another is a constantly sober and scientific explanation of this; and a third quality is Hoffmeyer's honest attempt to restrict human communicative characteristics to humans, and present communication at other biological levels in terms distinctive from such human abilities as thinking and choosing. The difference in objectification in the popular and the semiotic model is of significance beyond the mere semantic. The semiotic reference to interpretation of signs rather than intelligence and thinking is *"a difference, that makes a difference"* (to speak with Bateson), in so far as signs – as well as the interpretation of them – can be biochemical, i.e., without implying any mystical assumptions of intelligence or thinking on a biochemical level. The model of semiosis not only reformulates the notion of a non-mechanical human body and nature in semantic terms, but also reframes the signs by interpreting them as signs referring to communication in the body, and between body and environment, in a scientific frame of reference. Non-mechanical processes in cells, bodies and galaxies are no longer objectified in the image of man but within a scientific discourse of multilevel communication. In a semiotic model, this difference can be illustrated as in figure 3.

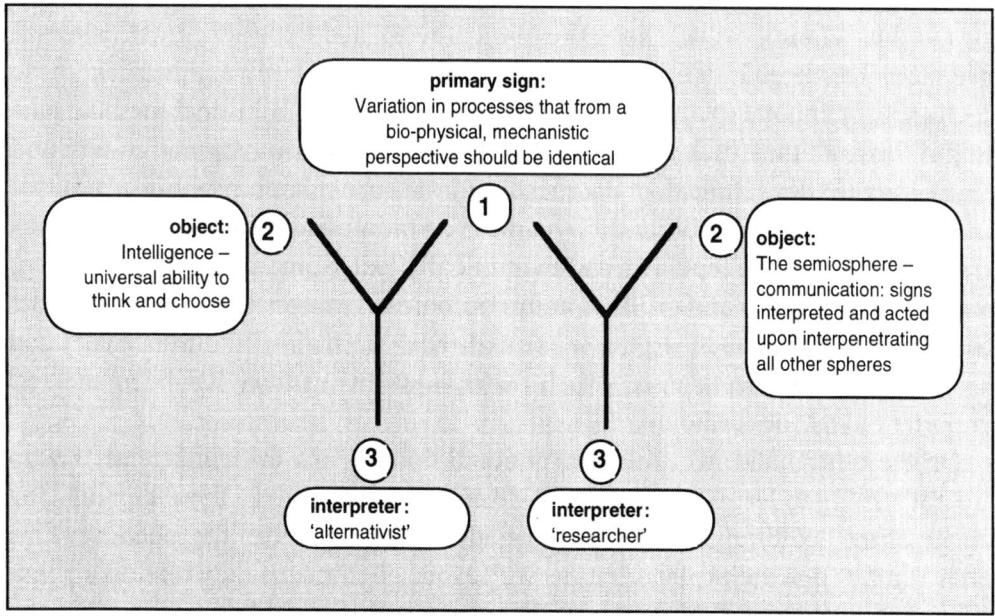

Figure 3

When the Doctor Goes Bananas

The two objectifications presented above refer to somewhat identical organizational and structural patterns in the world and, yet, they are quite different and most likely to evoke very different responses in different contexts.

The anthropomorphic image – in which the cell goes cultural – is likely to be meaningful to lay-people as it represents the world in well-known, homely terms. An ordinary "Mrs. Jones" can understand it, and it presents to her some logical explanations for that which cannot be explained in mechanical terms. To her, it makes sense that cells and bodies think and choose and, thus, react differently to identical stimuli. No matter how crazy this idea may seem to sceptics and conventional doctors, one must not oversee the significance of the image. It is highly meaningful to lay-people and provides the rationale to engage in happenings which may be helpful, though others would explain the whole thing differently. The clients of Ivor James found comfort and support for their daily life in the sittings. This was only possible as long as they could objectify the sittings within the popular cosmology. Most rejected James' explanation of the sittings, because that explanation did not make sense to them and, therefore, did not "work" for them. Those that believed him stopped coming, because withdrawn from the frame of popular cosmology the sittings did not "work" any more.

Quite interestingly, not only clients and lay-healers seem to accept and use anthropomorphic popular models of the body, sickness and healing. Such models are also promoted by several medical doctors who use alternative therapies in their clinical work. Since the clinical work and experience with alternative therapies exceed traditional medical models for the body and healing, these doctors just cannot explain their experiences within the traditional medical paradigm. Instead, they pick up explanations and models from popular culture and cosmology. When clinical phenomena cannot be explained within a physio-anatomical realm and monitored by simple counting and measurement, doctors are, by and large, conceptually and theoretically lost. Some are willing to accept popular explanations and produce anthropomorphic images of the world and the body. They "go bananas" in the sense that they "go native" ("alternative") and lose the grounding in science which throughout this century has been such an important ideal for medicine.

On the other hand, we find conventional doctors and critical scientists who are not willing to let go of the scientific basis of medicine. To these persons, the image of the "culturalized cell" is most annoying and blocks for meaning. This often implies that the explanations as well as the phenomena they refer to are dismissed as non-sense and of no significance. These people "go bananas" in the sense that they refuse to see the importance in the phenomena and respond to the whole thing in an aggressive, ridiculing way. In my opinion, these people throw out the baby with the bath water.

The point is that no matter how sceptical we are of the explanations, we do, after all, have to accept that *something* happens in alternative therapy. Multiple studies show that people get relieved at least in subjective terms. But we do not know how and why. The explanations offered by alternative therapists in general are not satisfactory for critical academics, but it seems possible to find academic models that could explain the observations. These models may not be widely used within medicine of today, but being scholarly based they may be relevant models for medicine of tomorrow.

My suggestion is that many phenomena in alternative therapy can be reformulated (reobjectified) within scientific frames of reference by looking beyond traditional medical science. In this paper I have suggested a model of biological semiosis as a substitute for the model of cells and molecules thinking and choosing. The model proposed is thoroughly based in the sciences of biology and biochemistry. It is not less cultural than the anthropomorphic image, but it refers to academic culture rather than to popular culture and may, therefore, be more suitable for academic discussions of alternative therapies.

There are, of course, multiple ways to reformulate alternative therapies within academic discourse. The above should more be considered an example than a final solution to such a reformulation. In another paper, I have tried to reframe whole treatment sessions from selected kinds of alternative therapy in an anthropological perspective. This reframing provides a reobjectification of the clinical encounter between alternative healers and their clients pointing to a potential therapeutic effectiveness of elements not usually considered part of the "treatment". My point is that alternative techniques of diagnosis can act as therapies in themselves. These techniques produce individual, holistic images of the patients and create conceptual patterns within which the chaos of sickness can become ordered and meaningful to the patients. Such cultural reordering of the sickness experience may imply potentials for improvement of the patients wellbeing, in the first place referring to the illness experience of patients, but – in the light of research within psycho-neuro-immunology – perhaps also secondarily and indirectly to the disease (the pathological disorder) (Johannessen 1996).

I am sure that many other models from biology, physics, anthropology, psychology etc., can substitute traditional alternative models and, thus, make the phenomena understandable for those who cannot accept the popular models. With a focus on communication in and about alternative therapies, I propose that discussions be based in a general recognition of the significance of communication for our conceptualization of phenomena (be it symptoms or whole treatment sessions). By recognizing this, we give room for diversity in explanatory models and need not waste our time on arguments of what is true and what is false. Rather, we can concentrate on the significance of this primary act of objectification for communication and relations between healers and patients or between doctors and healers. On behalf of Jesper Hoffmeyer's and others' work, we may also consider the importance of multi-level communication for non-mechanical processes in the body, sickness and healing.

Epilogue

During my conversation with Ivor James, he was drawing a picture which he gave to me at the end of the session. It was a picture of a woman's face, and I asked James who it was. He said that he did not know who it was but that I might think of it as a symbolic representation of helpful forces in the world. In continuation of this, he said that many people believed his drawings to represent a personal spiritual guide (be it a deceased relative, an American Indian or a Chinese sage). James himself did not believe spiritual guides to be human-like as indicated by the drawings. He did not believe spiritual guides to have any bodies or bodily appearances, but as he said, it would not work very well just to hand over a blank piece of paper while telling the client that this is a picture of her spiritual guide. The lay-client would not be able to understand and appreciate this, even though it might be more "true" in academic terms.

In spite of all my academic training and academic considerations, as presented above, I rather liked the drawing which James gave to me. I hang it just above my desk and even named the lady. I call her Eleanor, just because I think she looks like an Eleanor (I do not personally know any dead or living persons of that name). Every once in a while, when I get stuck in the middle of writing a paper (like this), I take a look at Eleanor and feel very good in knowing that she is with me. This very anthropomorphic representation of support for my work makes me feel safe and at home.

References

Hoffmeyer, Jesper
  1994   *En snegl på vejen. Betydningens naturhistorie,* Samlerens Bogklub: Copenhagen.

Johannessen, Helle
  1996   "Individualized Knowledge", in: S. Cant & U. Sharma (eds.): *Complementary Medicines; Knowledge in Practice,* Free Association Books: London (forthcoming).

Part III

Homoeopathy and Placebo

Building a Professional Community; Collective Culture in a Group of Non Medically Qualified Homoeopaths in Britain

by Ursula Sharma

The literature about professionalisation is full of references to 'strategies', 'projects' (e.g., Witz 1992). Yet who or what are the agents who entertain these projects, seek to carry out strategies? According to this literature they are groups of would-be professionals organised into associations which then act corporately on behalf of the emergent profession.

For an association to develop in the first place there must be networks of practitioners with established patterns of interaction and some sense of common cause. To develop effective strategies there needs to be some degree of consensus about means and ends, about how members communicate with each other and with agencies outside the profession, i.e., there must be some degree of common political culture, as well as common occupational skills and knowledge. I realise that the use of the term 'culture' in relation to organisations is contentious for anthropologists (see Case 1994). I am using it here simply as a convenient 'shorthand' way of referring to certain common forms of communication and ways of doing things which are pervasive and relatively persistent within a group. As we shall see, the origins of the 'cultural' practices which I shall identify may be fairly heterogeneous, some deliberately and self-consciously cultivated within the group, others imported from other social and cultural domains, as the various members of the emerging group come together to realise their commonalties, and (as we shall see) their differences.

The ways in which such cultures develop among professions has been given little attention. Where orthodox medicine is concerned, quite a lot of research has been done on the ways in which professional education helps to generate certain attitudes of mind (e.g., Becker et al. 1961, Good 1994). And prior to the experience of education there is the process of selection of candidates for that education. It has become evident that medical schools in Britain often chose candidates who conformed to certain norms – insistence on science 'A' level examination passes, preference for people with middle class background, possibly children of doctors, preference for male candidates, exclusion of foreigners (see

CRE 1988). Consciously or otherwise, prior to the introduction of equal opportunities policies (and possibly even then), they were selecting people who could be presumed to have a fair degree of cultural community already, excluding ethnic minorities, women, working class candidates, those with recent background in humanities etc.

Where complementary therapy in Britain is concerned, however, one of the major problems in unifying a community of practitioners so that a national organisation can be formed has been the divisive effect of training having been given in highly diverse establishments, often founded by influential and charismatic practitioners, with their own distinctive ethos and version of the therapy. Many of these training establishments had already set up professional associations exclusively for their own alumni, and sometimes it proved hard to integrate all these into one.

The Society of Homoeopaths, which I shall consider here, did not have this particular problem but originated in a group of people who had common experience of being taught informally by two influential and charismatic teachers in the late sixties and early seventies (Cant, forthcoming). I have conducted research on this organisation for several years, attending its conferences and gatherings, interviewing local members and officers and scanning its journals and publications. I present here some observations based on this fieldwork, concerning myself chiefly with the extent to which the Society can be said to have developed a common social and political culture.[1]

The Society of Homoeopaths; Historical Background

In Britain homoeopathy is practised by two main kinds of practitioner, doctor homoeopaths and non-medically qualified homoeopaths (NMQ homoeopaths).[2] The Faculty of Homoeopaths provides postgraduate training in homoeopathy for people who are already qualified in medicine. Until recently the courses provided by the Faculty constituted the only formal homoeopathic education available in Britain. In the seventies, two NMQ homoeopaths – John Da Monte and

---

1 Some of the interviews on which I have drawn in this paper were carried out by Sarah Cant as part of a wider project on the professionalisation of complementary medicine, funded by the Economic and Social Research Council. I acknowledge both this funding support and Sarah's practical and intellectual contribution to the development of my ideas. I also acknowledge the help of the Society itself in permitting the research and of those individual directors, administrators and members who gave specific help.
2 I use the term 'NMQ' in preference to the term 'lay', which as NMQ homoeopaths themselves point out, suggests a less than professional command of knowledge.

Thomas Maughan – taught groups of students, probably mostly ex-patients, in their homes. The two were friends, though their study groups were run separately. Da Monte had learnt most of what he knew about homoeopathy from Maughan himself and the latter seems to have learnt his homoeopathy informally from a member of the Faculty (see Morrell 1995 for a more detailed genealogy of NMQ homoeopathy in Britain). Homoeopathic knowledge therefore seems to have seeped out of the medical academy. In spite of these informal links, the doctor homoeopaths of the Faculty did not, and still do not, recognise the NMQ homoeopath as equal in competence to the doctor homoeopath. This exclusion, and the general contempt in which the medical profession as a body held practitioners of complementary medicine in general no doubt contributed to a sense of solidarity within the group, a sense of campaigning for the virtues of homoeopathy from a beleaguered position.

Da Monte and Maughan died within a few months of each other in 1975/6. The Society of Homoeopaths was founded by their pupils in 1978 to help encourage the development of NMQ homoeopathy in Britain, and a new college, the College of Homoeopathy, was founded in London in the same year, the first of a number of colleges founded by the pupils of Maughan and Da Monte. The only other association of NMQ homoeopaths had its origin in a more direct leakage from medical homoeopathy. Its members were mainly drawn from graduates of the Hahnemann College of Homoeopathy, founded by an Indian doctor, Dr. Pyara Singh, in 1980 and staffed mainly by medically qualified doctors. This college provides training mainly, though not exclusively, for people who have some professional qualification in a field such as nursing or dentistry. The United Kingdom Homeopathic Medical Association was founded in 1985, originally primarily as a professional association for graduates of the Hahnemann College, though it is now open to graduates of other colleges as well.

These two organisations started out quite separately and with rather different kinds of membership and orientation, although there has been a good deal of rapprochement in recent years, and some considerable overlap of membership. However, what made the Society of Homoeopaths quite distinct, and the factor which has shaped a good deal of its development (though some would say has caused it problems), was the fact that both Da Monte and Maughan were active Druids, also keenly interested in esoteric and Eastern philosophy, and they evidently mixed these interests in their teaching of homoeopathy to their pupils in the late sixties and seventies. (Druids are members of a revived esoteric pagan order, famous for their gathering at the prehistoric sacred site of Stonehenge at the summer solstice). It is not quite clear to me exactly how this took place – I have the impression that the issue of Druidism generally seems to be perceived as something of a potential embarrassment among a group of people now committed to the professional development of NMQ homoeopathy, with state registration as a realistic ambition.

As one founder member of the Society recalled in an interview:

> "Several of us became Druids though we did not keep it up for terribly long after Maughan died. You know we went to Stonehenge for the equinox and the summer solstice for the ceremony there. It was quite fun. My son also put on a sort of costume sheet and all three of us carried this heavy cross. We were there all night doing this sort of vigil and it was quite an experience".

This kind of activity may be recalled with amused nostalgia, but the writings of the pupils of Da Monte make clear that many of the founder members of the Society of Homoeopaths (and indeed many who have more recently joined) continue to regard healing as being not at all divorced from spiritual issues in the broad sense. Homoeopathic treatment is seen as a possible means of developing personal awareness and potential, not just a means for treating symptoms.

I know very little about the cultural background of the pupils of Da Monte and Maughan, or their experience prior to learning homoeopathy, so it is difficult to say how much of what I identify as the cultural atmosphere of the Society and its meetings and activities might be regarded as the specific outcome of their experiences as students, or as stemming more generally from the ethos of the social milieu in which they grew up, the general ambience of the sixties etc. And in any case, these founder members are not the only influential individuals in the Society as it has grown and developed, although for some years the majority of directors and office holders were former pupils of Da Monte and Maughan.

Forms of Communication; Intimacy and Informality

So much for historical background. Let me now share a few impressions.

When I attended the annual conference of the Society in 1991 the welcoming speech was given by one of the directors of the Society. At the end he asked us all to stand up and turn to our right. We were then to give our neighbour a light neck massage, to relieve any stiffness people might feel after making the long journey to the conference venue, and to break the ice. People did this with some amusement but (it would seem) little embarrassment. The presentations which followed were very varied in style and content, but in general the mode of delivery was informal. Some speakers gave very interactive presentations, asking questions of the audience (the patient had such and such symptoms, what remedy do you think the homoeopath should suggest?). This latter device seems to be a regular stylistic feature of the kind of homoeopathic seminars attended and given by members of the Society, with the audience frequently being invited to name the remedies they would give in a case, invited (as it were) to participate in the process of reasoning being described in an account of a case.

Few speakers at the conference read from notes, and some gave presentations that seemed rather *ex tempore* to me, though not necessarily rambling or inconclusive. I noted that the style of dress favoured by the speakers, and indeed most of the participants, was what might be called smart casual, or even just casual – few suits, but at the same time, few denims either.

This general theme of informality and intimacy is often manifested in written communications of the Society. In the newsletter well known homoeopaths are often referred to by first names, and the letter column contains much first name reference also.

The informality I noticed may derive from the personal intimacy among the founding group but could also be related to the image Society homoeopaths have of themselves as professionals who aim for a less hierarchical relationship with patients (opposed to their perception of orthodox medical relations). Whilst osteopaths favour white coats when seeing patients (perhaps useful as a distancing device in a therapy which involves touching the patient, a patient often in a state of undress?), homoeopaths, as I have observed, do not favour uniforms or 'power dressing' of any kind, rather a style of dress which is unlikely to distance them from patients. Here, however, one of the ambiguities in the sense of what it is to be a professional surfaced when a student whom I met related that he had been told by his tutor that his style of dress was rather untidy (indeed the fact was noted in his end of year report) and that, as an aspiring professional, he should come to college rather more smartly dressed. This encapsulates a contradiction which the Society faces on a number of fronts; on the one hand, Society homoeopaths have explicitly rejected the symbols of power and distance which they associate with those aspects of orthodox medicine which they dislike. On the other hand, in as much as they aspire to state registration and more formal legitimation as a profession, they are under some pressure to conform to what they think the public expects in a serious professional – a certain degree of smartness and conventional formality.

Communication Again; Styles of Humour

I often wonder why anthropologists study humour as little as they do. They are

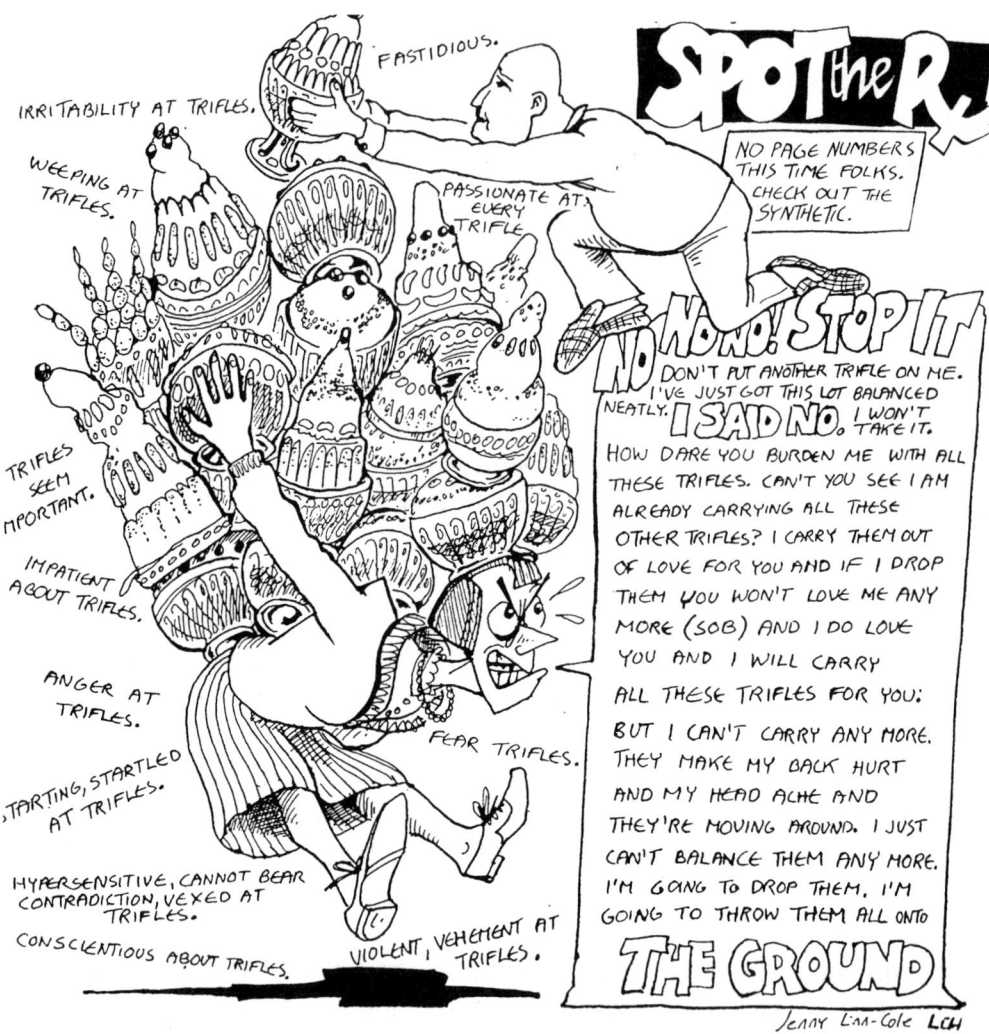

'Cartoon which originally appeared on the cover of the newsletter of the Society of Homoeopaths, June 1993. I am grateful to the Society for kindly allowing me to reproduce it here'.

not a humourless breed, but they seldom tell us much about the kind of jokes which a particular group find funny.

Yet humour is an important dimension of the common culture and identity of a group. A few studies have been made of humour in the workplace, the way in which it can express both solidarities and exclusions (e.g., Sykes 1966). One use of humour which I noted at conferences and other public events was jocular use of the language of the repertory,[3] along the lines of (on a very hot day) 'those who are suffering from air, lack of, and think they are suffocating, may like to take a break outside before the next session'.

In fact the repertory and the *materia medica* of homoeopathy are good sources of humour, as the cartoon reproduced here (meant to depict particular remedy profiles) indicates. Note that the interactive device I mentioned in connection with seminars is also used (the reader is invited to guess the remedy).

I am not arguing that homoeopaths have a sense of humour which is essentially different from that of other professional groups, though this may be the case. Homoeopathic joking however is based on insider knowledge; it refers to knowledge which is otherwise taken very seriously indeed. Homoeopaths are allowed to mock their own knowledge as a means of expressing their common identity, much as a Jewish comedian may make a Jewish joke which might be construed as anti-Semitic or tasteless were it recounted by anyone else.

Developing a Political Culture; Basic Assumptions and Styles of Action

To develop a project and to pursue it consistently, the members of an association must already share to some extent, or else must develop, a political culture. By this I do not mean that they must actually agree on all political matters, simply that they must share some dominant values and notions about the proper way to go about getting things done, including the right way to resolve disagreements. The Society of Homoeopaths, like many similar professional organisations in the field of complementary medicine, has had to make the transition from a coterie of inspired activists to a formally constituted public group, capable of being taken seriously as a proper professional association, with all that this implies in terms of being capable of enforcing ethical codes, guarantee competence of registered members etc. On the whole it has done this remarkably rapidly and successfully, with the founder members evidently conscious of the need to both develop stable and appropriate management structures, yet also harness the enthusiasm of a 'second wave' generation of activists – many of them their own former pupils.

---

3 The homoeopathic 'repertory' is a compilation of symptoms, ordered largely according to the various parts of the body. For example, an entry in Kent's widely used repertory is as follows: in the 'Abdomen' section we have subheadings referring to sensations such as: Loose, as if intestines were; Lump, in abdomen, sensation of; Menses, would appear, sensation as if; and in the 'Mind' section we have a heading: Talk, indisposed to; and subheadings such as: air, in open; alternating with quarrelsomeness; eating, after. With each symptomatic entry there is a list of possible remedies.

The Society has a formal constitution which gives a good deal of discretion to an elected Board of between six and nine Directors. With the growth of membership and functions the Directors initiated a review of management in 1992 which resulted in (amongst other things) the setting up of various working groups dealing with specialised areas, to which ordinary members were invited to offer their services (Society of Homoeopaths Newsletter June 1993: 8). The Society certainly sees itself explicitly as 'non-hierarchical and democratic' (Society of Homoeopaths Newsletter March 1994: 5). In spite of periodic complaints from members that the Directors are 'remote' from the ordinary membership, the Directors seem to have worked hard at developing regular channels of communication between the officers and the ordinary membership. Possibly some members have found this regular trawling for the experiences and opinions of membership has gone a bit too far, as this humourous comment delivered in the context of a cabaret show at the annual conference suggests:

"May you never be selected for a Society questionnaire
May you never find there's headlice in your hair
May you never find your pimples turn into a scabies spot
May you never sneeze out Kali Bichrom[4] snot"
(Society of Homoeopaths Annual Report 1994: inside back cover).

On the whole there appears to have been few fundamental disagreements about the constitution of the Society and its formal working (I am not speaking here of substantive differences about how homoeopathy itself should be practised or taught, of which there have been a few, some quite important). However, from a number of sources (comments made in interviews, letters and articles in the Society Newsletter etc.) one picks up certain underlying political tensions, or perhaps one should say ambivalences. These are not to do with the organisation of the Society as such, but they do surface in relation to particular issues which the Society has to tackle. These are in the nature of felt contradictions between different but related goals rather than conflicts between identified factions or groups of people.

For example, there is the anxiety which was, and to some extent still is, frequently voiced in the complementary therapy movement (not just among homoeopaths) between the need to professionalise in order to be 'respectable' and accepted, and the fear that once NMQ practitioners become a profession they will

---

4 *Kali Bichromicum* is a homoeopathic remedy which, according to one *materia medica*, is associated with such symptoms as 'discharge (from nose) thick, ropy, greenish yellow. Tough elastic plugs from nose'.

act in the self-serving way attributed to the medical profession, losing their idealism. Statutory regulation is widely held to be an important goal for NMQ homoeopaths. Yet Pauline Price, herself a doctor studying to become a homoeopath, voices the worry that whilst homoeopaths ought to be striving for a professional approach to their work,

> "Devious means can be used to achieve a given end. Concern can be professed for the people when the profession is really self-serving. So the danger of a profession is that its members become self-serving" (Society of Homoeopaths Newsletter December 1995: 13).

Secondly, there is the tension between an ethos of cooperation and mutual support in a beleaguered group, and the realisation that once the supply of homoeopaths reaches a certain level, practitioners are actually competing with each other for a living in a market which is not unlimited. (This is a problem for many complementary practitioners, not just homoeopaths; see Sharma 1995: 159.) On the one hand, members of the Society have worked hard at building up local networks of homoeopaths who provide support for each other and share information. On the other, the directorate has had to recognise that from the patient's point of view the various homoeopaths in an area are in competition for his/her patronage; what etiquette should be inscribed into the code of ethics to deal with the situation when a patient transfers from one homoeopath to another (Society of Homoeopaths Newsletter September 1993: 3)?

To illustrate the way in which such emergent tensions have surfaced, I will describe only one such issue in detail, that of gender equality.

Gender and the Political Culture of the Society

A feature of the Society's meetings which I noticed very early on was the predominance of women. This reflects the composition of the membership at the present time (less than a third of the 360 odd registered members are men, a gender imbalance which seems to be reproduced in the current student body also, judging by class lists of homoeopathic colleges which I have come across). Whether as a cause or a consequence of this 'feminisation' of the professional group, there seems a fair degree of gender consciousness reflected in publications and activities. A creche is a regular feature of the conference and larger gatherings. In January 1980 a note in the Newsletter announced that an explanatory leaflet produced earlier was being revised so that all reference to 'he' was being replaced by 'he or she' throughout when both sexes were intended, and other publications of the Society from about this time reflect a strong consciousness of the need to avoid sexist language (although a more radical and innovative attempt to devise a gender-neutral pronoun in the annual reports was abandoned as too divergent from ordinary speech practice).

More controversial was the decision to hold women only conferences, the first of several being held in 1991. A letter to the Society's Newsletter from one of the participants hailed the conference as a useful new departure which would do something to redress the disproportionate practical dominance of men in the Society (disproportionate that is in relation to the feminine nature of the membership already remarked upon). This letter produced uncomprehending responses in the following issue from two other members, who evidently could not see the necessity for a women only conference when women actually predominated in the Society, and felt uncomfortable about what they perceived as a too militant style of ensuring gender equality:

> "I, being a person first and also a woman, don't want to be included as a participant in a crusading march and banner parade to save downtrodden Homoeopathic womanhood – no such thing really exists in this country".

And from a (male) founder member:

> "Is it only a matter of numbers?. . . I would like to divert the talk about male/female numbers on the Board of Directors to that of suitability for the job" (Society of Homoeopaths Newsletter 31, 1991).

The women's conference seems to have become an accepted feature of the Society year in spite of this reaction, and the controversy consequent upon this first conference was to become drowned in a wider controversy that broke out over the nature of homoeopathic prescribing, which was to prove far more divisive. However, the incident is worth mentioning to illustrate the fact that common commitment to homoeopathy and broadly similar cultural background does not in itself ensure that the members of an emergent professional group have the same ideas about the kind of political practices that are normal and acceptable, or the kind of political language which should be used within the group. As I see it, the debate about the women's conference was not about substantive issues (are women or men better homoeopaths, more worthy to be directors etc?) but about political method and style – tension between a basically liberal position (stressing individual identity; 'we can have equal opportunities without feminism – gender identity is unimportant, and we should not divide the movement') and a more radical position affected by practice of creating 'women only' spaces used in a number of other contexts by feminists. Some women were more comfortable than others with what they saw as a 'militant' style of action, although the positions and method taken by the more feminist members were far from 'extreme' and the public disagreement was on the whole relatively muted.

The Emergent Profession; Colleges and Networks

The emerging public culture of the group as I have described it so far is based on a number of ingredients: the familiarity and friendship which obtained among the founding group and is reproduced among cohorts of new students, the solidarity engendered through the perception of being a threatened group, some deliberate decisions made as a matter of public relations policy with regard to style and design of publications, members' notions about the kind of profession homoeopaths should aspire to be and about the proper way to achieve it, their ideas and feelings about different styles of activism and their experiences of activism in other contexts.

In the end the dominant and enduring culture of NMQ homoeopathy will be made primarily in the colleges. Common experience of training (whatever the form it takes) with its rites of passage, its trials and solidarities, is an important basis for the formation of professional identity – whether we are dealing with healing professions or any other.

Professional education is more than the ingestion of certain information required to do professional work. It involves the adoption of certain ways of thinking and communicating and interacting with others through the practices of the professional academy, whatever the nature of that academy may be. Thus, Good describes how medical students at Harvard learn medicine through the acquisition of a particular way of constructing the human body, learnt through experiences such as the dissection of a cadaver, use of slides in lectures etc. (Good 1994: 73).

They also learn certain forms of communication, such as the writing up of case notes. A student tells him:

> "The ideal write-up has all the facts that argue in favour and all the facts that argue against, and conclusions drawn from those ... drawn together in a sort of summarizing formulation about what you think is going on, and then a plan of attack.... There is something very satisfying about that. ... You begin to approach the patient now with a write-up in mind. To a large extent you are authorized through your writing" (Good 1994: 77).

A good write-up of a case establishes the student as someone who has learnt what is relevant to pick out from the interview, experienced as an event, to communicate to colleagues and to put on the record.

I do not have the kind of material on homoeopathic education that Good gathered on biomedical education since, whilst I have interviewed both school principals and recently graduated homoeopaths, I never interviewed students themselves. However, from interviews with recent graduates, study of material put out by colleges etc., we can get some hints.

The founding generation of homoeopaths created a group culture based on the way they had developed as a very informal group of friends and fellow students. Informality still seems to be a characteristic of education with the frequent use of forenames which I noted earlier. Most of the original group is still involved in homoeopathic education in some way. Many founded colleges of which they are now principals, and there is much mutual visiting; members of the original group often give guest lectures in each others' colleges, and act as each others' external examiners.

Most colleges work with small groups, largely because they are still relatively small institutions. However, smallness and intimacy have also been perceived as a positive virtue by some educators. One school even called itself for some time the Small School of Homoeopathy (as in 'small is beautiful' – I thought at first it had been founded by a person with the surname of Small). But whilst professionalisation does not require size, it does require a degree of formalisation of the educational process, if only in the sense that a respectable professional course must have recognised forms of validation, transparent criteria for assessment of performance, a proper system of external examiners etc. Interviews with college principals showed that whilst the impetus for this kind of development came as much from the educators as anyone else in the homoeopathic world, they did not always find it easy to move from the informal/charismatic mode of transmission of knowledge through discipleship to the formal/bureaucratic mode of the publicly legitimated modern professional academy. Many were concerned as to how they should move to the latter without losing some of the inspiration and personal care they saw as characteristic of the former.

Another salient aspect of homoeopathic education is that it is largely part-time at the moment. The students are mature men and women (mostly the latter) who have typically had some other career. That is, they will already have been inducted into some other profession before coming to homoeopathy; they are less 'raw material' than the typical medical student who proceeds straight to training from high school, and their sense of professional identity will not be forged in the same way. They prepare to be homoeopaths by attending courses of (usually) four years, studying intensively at monthly weekend sessions. On the other hand, it is a very different kind of educational experience from that described by the medical students whom Good studied, in as much as the students are not cut off and immersed in their academy; it is not a 'total experience'. Medical school

" . . . is a forced emotional experience. We handle cadavers, we have faeces labs, where we examine our own faeces, go to mental hospital where we get locked up with screaming patients. These are total experiences like an occult thing or a boot camp . . . Its not just an extension of college. College was also a total experience but you get by with much less direct engagement. I feel like I am changing my brain every day, moulding it in a specific way" (Good 1994: 65).

Homoeopathic educators do not have the opportunity at the present time to offer this kind of 'bush initiation' experience to their students, who remain heavily exposed during the entirety of their course to non-homoeopathic definitions of illness, and the non-homoeopathic world in general.

Nonetheless, from what some former students have told me, it would seem that the sense of solidarity which develops among a cohort of students is very strong. A number of colleges have student journals, produced by the students themselves, which incidentally seem to demonstrate much the same kind of cultural ethos as the public output of the Society itself – circle dancing, tepee building and rambling were more likely to be publicised in the small advertisements and news pages than, say, squash ladders, and there was the same first-name intimacy with reference to both staff and students.

A good number of graduates evidently enter into professional cooperation of one kind or another with former classmates, perhaps in the form of some kind of joint practice. Setting up in practice on one's own is often a very difficult and isolating experience and the Society has recognised the need for ongoing professional contact through support groups, or local supervision groups, in which an established homoeopath holds sessions for recently graduated homoeopaths practising in a certain area to come together, discuss problems and seek advice on specific cases. The relative structural isolation of the homoeopathic student or the newly qualified homoeopath is therefore balanced by existence of informal regional or local networks which mostly have an established homoeopath at their centre.

The shape of the collective professional culture and community that emerges will depend much on the ethos of the colleges, the kind of interaction favoured between staff and students, the kind of values and attitudes cultivated in students. What I have been able to give here is only a rather tentative sketch of the kinds of considerations which might prove important. It would be interesting for an anthropologist to conduct the same kind of study of homoeopathic education as Good and Becker have done for orthodox medicine.

Concluding Remarks

I have dealt with styles of communication and interaction rather than the substantive issues which homoeopaths communicate about or the details of the formal politics of the group. I have not touched upon debates about classical versus 'not-so-classical' homoeopathic prescribing, debates about the structure of the Society, or the nature of homoeopathic education. Rather, I have concentrated on the informal and the implicit, the apparently trivial and the assumed . . . but as any anthropologist will tell you, it is these apparently trivial aspects of everyday communication which you notice when you come into another culture – most of the time the members of the group do not have to notice it; it is part of the cultural air they breathe, and as such is as important to communication and solidarity as air is to life.

References

Becker, H., Geer, B., Hughes, E. and Strauss, L.
1961 *Boys in White: Student Culture in Medical School,* Chicago University Press: Chicago.

Case, P.
1994 "Tracing the organisational culture debate", in: *Anthropology in Action*, 1(2): 9-12.

Cant, S. (forthcoming)
"From charismatic teaching to professional training: the legitimation of knowledge and the creation of trust" in: S. Cant and U. Sharma (eds.): *Complementary Medicines; Knowledge in Practice,* Free Association Books: London.

Commission for Racial Equality
1988 *Admissions to Medical Schools*, Commission for Racial Equality: London.

Good, B.
1994 *Medicine, Rationality and Experience. An Anthropological Perspective,* Cambridge University Press: Cambridge.

Maceoin, D.
1993 "The choice of homoeopathic models: the patient's dilemma", in: *The Homoeopath*, 51: 108-115.

Morrell, P.
1995 "A brief history of British lay homoeopathy", in: *The Homoeopath*, 59: 471-5.

Sharma, U.
1995 *Complementary Medicine Today. Practitioners and Patients*, Routledge: London.

Sykes, A.
1966 "Joking relationships in an industrial setting", in: *American Anthropologist*, 62: 188-193.

Witz, A.
1992 *Professions and Patriarchy*, Routledge: London.

A Hearing for Homoeopathy: Some Sociological Reflections on Problems of Communication about Alternative Therapy among Researchers and Practitioners

by Phillip Nicholls

Among the great variety of alternative or (for those of a less radical disposition) complementary therapies which are now available to the discerning consumer of health care, homoeopathy has one of the longest pedigrees. Throughout its history, it has also had a chronic problem of communication. It has to be admitted that Samuel Hahnemann, homoeopathy's founding figure, was himself responsible for helping to ensure that things began as they would continue as far as communication with the medical world was concerned: He was not shy of advertising his own infallibility, or of belittling his erstwhile therapeutic colleagues, neither of which activities did much to incline his audience to listen with a dispassionate ear to his ideas. Indeed, the trade in insults between homoeopaths and regular practitioners became a pastime which medical men seem to have adopted with increasing vigour during the first three quarters of the nineteenth century.

This period in homoeopathy's turbulent career introduces the role of occupational and status interests, which is the first of five themes which I want, rather eclectically, to examine in terms of developing a sociological understanding of the factors involved in inhibiting (or enhancing) communication about alternative therapy. The second theme concerns the connection between a resurgence of interest in complementary therapy and aspects of the so-called postmodern condition. It will be argued that certain changes have occurred in the structure and culture of societies which have helped to facilitate an interest in the irregular and the unorthodox. Three other aspects of the postmodern condition – the stabilisation of identity in a world of flux, impermanence and change, the focus on consumption, and the emphasis on the body – form the third theme. The point here will be that in so far as problems of identity may be resolved either through the social practice of knowledge systems (such as homoeopathy etc.), or through the consumption of them, then the scientific interrogation of these systems can also be seen to involve a challenge to 'the self'.

The fourth theme focuses on the problems of communication among different therapists which may ensue when concepts of health and of the body, as constructed within one discourse (homoeopathy say, or acupuncture), are incommensurable with their construction in another, such as that of scientific medicine. The way in which different discourses compete in order to establish the legitimacy of their particular therapeutic paradigm forms the basis of the fifth and final theme. Using a particular case study – that of the Bristol Cancer Help Centre in the UK – the processes involved in the social construction and defence of biomedical orthodoxy in cancer treatment are highlighted, and the role of medical journals in ensuring the reproduction and communication of 'legitimate' and 'objective' knowledge emphasized.

Returning now, however, to the themes raised in my opening paragraphs: how can the acrimonious dialogue between homoeopaths and allopaths best be understood in the nineteenth century? An examination of these exchanges in Britain and in the USA (Nicholls 1988) shows that, with one or two exceptions, the doctors involved were talking *past* each other, rather than *to* each other. Much more energy was expended in trading vitriol, slur and character assassination than in attempts to shed light on the issue that supposedly divided the two schools: whether or not reasonable evidence could be gathered which would suggest that patients treated homoeopathically fared better (or worse) than those treated by conventional means, or not treated at all. Indeed, the striking thing is that, with the sole exception of a trial of homoeopathic remedies in veterinary practice (Nicholls 1988: 153-4), no investigation into the comparative effectiveness of the two systems appears to have been carried out at all in Britain during this period. To be sure, homoeopaths and allopaths regularly threw statistics at each other, based on the therapeutic records of their own hospitals, but these were just another form of insult: neither side ever convinced the other for the rather obvious reason that the data was seen as manifestly suspicious.

What helped to produce this peculiar situation was the fact that the struggle between the two schools was really a struggle about medical incomes, and about the right to control the division of labour and the nature of training and practice within medicine. It needs to be remembered that, as far as Britain was concerned, the occupation of medicine in the first part of the nineteenth century was, in terms of prospective rewards, a dismal one. There were too many general practitioners, their incomes and level of public esteem were low, they were usually subject to lay authority by Boards of Governors of hospitals or by Poor Law administrators, and their interests were largely ignored by the elite physicians and surgeons of the Royal Colleges (see among many authors on this, Peterson 1978). In short, it was an occupational group whose ordinary members rapidly acquired a sense of collective interest, and which equally rapidly, under the impetus of radical reformers like Thomas Wakley, saw those interests as being realised through a process of professionalisation, which would help to regulate entry to medical work, raise educational standards and enhance the remuneration and prestige of doctors.

In these circumstances it was small wonder that those doctors who, by becoming homoeopaths, encouraged public scepticism of medical expertise, criticised their erstwhile allopathic colleagues, and who built prosperous and fashionable practices by weaning patients away from those of their rivals, were not about to be given the courtesy of a polite hearing for their particular therapeutic opinions. In accordance with this view, homoeopathic doctors in Britain and the USA found themselves dismissed from hospital posts, refused consultation rights and ostracised from medical associations and societies.

Occupational interests, then, in so far as they are articulated to the economic privileges of practice based on particular forms of knowledge, are likely to function in a way which protects those interests by subverting, distorting or silencing rival claims or systems. Indeed, this is probably as true today as it was in the nineteenth century, as my closing remarks on the Bristol Cancer Help Centre will try to demonstrate.

Homoeopathy, of course, did decline towards the end of the nineteenth century. The reasons for this are quite complex, with some authors (such as Rothstein 1972) emphasizing the impact of the scientific revolution in medicine, while others (for example, Coulter 1977) point to a combination of 'loss of faith' in homoeopathy by its practitioners, leading them to make too many therapeutic compromises (resulting in the homogenization of practice), and the undermining of homoeopathic education by a strategic alliance of the American Medical Association and corporate medical interests. Whatever the reasons, it is also clear that, at least as far as Britain was concerned, homoeopathy, instead of initiating a vigorous struggle to arrest or reverse decline, seemed rather (with a few polite noises of hurt protest) to withdraw gracefully into a secluded and comfortable retirement.

To understand this involves, I would argue, thinking (somewhat paradoxically) about the semiotics of consumption. From the beginning, homoeopathy was associated with the social elites and the aristocracy and royalty of Europe. It is interesting to speculate on the reasons for this. One factor may be that the public endorsement of homoeopathy, and the patronage of its doctors, was a way of indicating *status group membership* (Weber 1922). Homoeopathy was a potent symbol here, since the display of extravagant expenditure on the consumption of an infinitesimal dose was an excellent way of demonstrating social standing, and of belonging to that stratum of society where wealth made ordinary economic calculations and considerations redundant.

If this is true, then it helps to explain the complacent attitude of members of the British Homoeopathic Society (BHS) – which, at the time, consisted of no more than 200 doctors – towards the national decline of homoeopathy from the fourth quarter of the nineteenth century onwards. Quite simply, I suggest that for these practitioners the display of exclusive status group relationships was more important than political mobilisation and public campaigning on behalf of homoeopathy. Many of them were wealthy because of elite patronage, and were content that the consumption of homoeopathic medicine should remain a mark of social distinction and exclusivity.

Such at least seems to have been the view of Dr. John Henry Clarke who, frustrated at the apparent complacency of his colleagues, left the BHS in 1900 never to rejoin. Anxious that homoeopathy would atrophy, and that homoeopathic skills would be lost to medicine if wider public interest and patronage were not cultivated, Clarke began more or less systematically (and in opposition to the views of his colleagues) to train lay practitioners. For Clarke, the therapeutic potential of homoeopathy was the thing which really needed preservation; its social connotations were an irrelevant distraction as far as he was concerned. One of Clarke's pupils and protégés, J. Ellis Barker, echoed his sentiments. An important figure in the lay movement in Britain in the 1930s and 1940s, Barker (1932) scorned the BHS (and its counterpart of lay supporters, the British Homoeopathic Association) as nothing more than places where rich gentlemen could indulge in idle chatter.

The careers of Dr. Clarke and of Ellis Barker are only intelligible when set in the context of an era of retreat and decline for homoeopathy. In an increasingly scientific age, homoeopathy appeared more and more as an ossified relic of the past, as a system of medicine which had nothing to offer to the new generations of doctors and medical scientists. And, with the establishment of the National Health Service (NHS), which provided care free at the point of consumption, it seemed that homoeopathy's precipitous decline might be terminal. Why, after all, should ordinary people pay for homoeopathic treatment from lay practitioners when their local general practitioner and hospital were funded by the government? True enough, the Faculty of Homoeopathy (as the BHS had become) was able – not least through its royal patronage – to preserve its place within the NHS, but it was very much a token presence, and its doctors continued to look to lucrative and select private practice rather than the public sector for financial reward.

Today, however, the picture is very different. Homoeopathy, along with other therapies, has experienced a quite dramatic renascence. Training courses for doctors offered by the Faculty of Homoeopathy are now, according to one recent in-house journal, "... *bursting at the seams*" (Clarke 1994: 138), while the lay movement now boasts some twenty training colleges in the UK, and the number of students, graduates and regular and associate members of the Society of Homoeopaths (the professional society of lay practitioners) had reached about 2,000 by the end of the 1980s (Society of Homoeopaths 1981-94).

What has created this climate where doctors and their patients are now willing to listen to alternative practitioners? A simple, popular rejection of the impersonal, technological and iatrogenic aspects of scientific medicine is certainly part of the explanation. Linked with this is probably the growth of ecological consciousness, and (ironically) the long period of hegemony of the New Right in politics, with its insistence on personal responsibility – a message which echoes the claim of many alternative practitioners that individuals in some sense 'choose' or 'deserve' their illnesses.

A more overarching explanation, however, might be embedded within the features claimed for the postmodern condition. For Lyotard (1984), this is characterised by (among other things) a fundamental loss of faith in the 'metanarrative of rationality' which has underpinned the modern age. Whether expressed as the ability of science or of universalising political philosophies to engineer a progressive liberation of humanity, this loss of faith has been driven by, for example, the continued presence of war, famine, global poverty, environmental degradation, genocide, the threat of nuclear holocaust, and the corruption and collapse of the great emancipatory project of Marxism.

The implications of this loss of faith in the ability of scientific rationality to work for universal human betterment are obvious enough as far as medicine is concerned. Here, too, much that seemed to have been promised as the fruit of scientific advance has not materialised: heart disease, stroke and cancer continue to evade successful medical intervention; new and powerful diseases, such as AIDS, continue to appear; bacteria have become resistant to antibiotics; and hospital wards produce infection and drug treatment new complications.

Scientific rationality, whatever form its substantive expression takes, is thereby shown, according to the postmodern argument, to have an unwarranted reputation for delivering either progress or enlightenment. The claim to universal validity – foundationalism – no longer has substance. In a world where Reason has failed there is room instead for many different voices. The postmodern condition, then, has created a climate where alternative therapies can speak and be heard.

A further aspect of the post or, if you are Anthony Giddens (1991), the *late* modern condition, is the so-called 'crisis of identity'. This introduces my third theme: the way in which selfhood may become involved in the process of communication about alternative therapies.

Postmodernity has created a crises of identity, so it is argued, because the traditional sources of validation for the self – class, neighbourhood, community and family – are dissolving. Furthermore, the body itself, once an apparently immutable haven of security for the embodied self, is now also a malleable resource as far as identity is concerned. Plastic surgery, implants, transplants, genetic manipulation, body building, diet and fitness regimes all testify to the ability to shape or choose the physical self. Even skin colour and sex are open to transformation.

The point, then, is that from a situation where 'the self' was given or fixed by an individual's particular location in the social structure, many people are now in a position to choose and change identities. (While I feel there is much in this claim I would, however, wish to enter a qualification: the 'project of the self' is only an option for those with the resources to pursue it – the constraints of class or, in perhaps its new manifestation, of *underclass* membership, are not so easily dismissed).

However, it does seem to be true that, for many people, identity is now something which it is possible to construct through the exercise of controlled choice in the sphere of consumption. The result of this activity is the use of products in a way which presents the self as an embodied text which can be read semiotically by others. Neither should we lose sight of the fact that this activity, although calculated, is not without its own inherent attraction: consumption can be straightforwardly hedonistic, pleasurable and sensual.

For alternative therapy the upshot of all this is that, as Professors McGuire (1995) and Spickard (1995) pointed out at the second INRAT conference, one solution which some people have clearly found to the problem of identity formation is the construction of the self as 'healer' or 'therapist'. In the sphere of consumption, many others may be choosing alternative therapies as a way of making a social statement about themselves. For both the producers and consumers of alternative therapy, then, more may be involved in the provision or use of treatment than its technical efficacy or possible *modus operandi*. In each case, personal meanings also seem to be at stake: for the therapist, the delivery of the treatment may also be the production of the self; for the consumer, the choice of therapy and of therapist may also be a way, as Jørgen Andersen (1995) has also pointed out, of sustaining a particular identity, reflecting a social status and (perhaps) of celebrating the sheer enjoyment of consumption. (One thinks of therapies involving movement, touch, talk and relaxation, for example, or of the rather obvious sensuality of treatments like aromatherapy).

In this way to communicate about alternative therapies with healers and their patients is seen to entail more than communication about knowledge, practice and technique: it is also a dialogue with the self, and may therefore, in certain cases, be interpreted as a hostile attempt to destabilize or renegotiate identity.

Just as the presence of the self may distort attempts to communicate between different kinds of healers, then a further difficulty emerges when the nature of health itself, or of the body as an object of therapeutic discourse, is constructed differently. This is a straightforward enough point, and need not detain us long.

Many alternative therapists construe health as more than the absence of disease. Instead, it is often seen as a *positive* emotional, psychological and physical sense of well-being which treatment can help to cultivate. Although this may have the unfortunate effect of creating a new army of the 'worried well', it is not actually such a very different idea to the currently fashionable 'lifestyle approach' to health advocated by many conventional practitioners. More serious problems seem to occur, however, when we compare the *body* as recognised and discussed by regular practitioners with its construction in terms of, say, homoeopathic discourse, or traditional Chinese acupuncture. Here, some fairly obvious difficulties soon emerge in terms of establishing common ground on which communication can take place. For homoeopaths, the patient's body is really nothing more than a collection of symptoms. Indeed, because of the 'law of similars', homoeopaths are actually much more at home in talking about the characteristics of remedies than in articulating conceptions of the body itself. Thus, while a medically trained practitioner would discuss, say, a disease process or entity as it impacted on body tissues, a homoeopath would talk about the remedy matched by the individual patient's symptoms. The two paradigms at work here construct the body very differently. They would, in fact, appear to be incommensurable. The same would appear to be true of those therapies, like traditional Chinese medicine, where the body is seen more in terms of energy flows and balances than organ and tissue systems.

Yet, given the increasing extent to which doctors and other kinds of healers work in a complementary way, dialogue *does* seem to succeed. It is already clear that one way in which this has been achieved is in terms of analogy (for example, the law of similars and action of potentised remedies in terms of the operation of the immune system), or by laboratory demonstration that techniques such as acupuncture are able to produce physiological responses recognisable and measurable in terms of conventional medicine. But this is a difficult and fascinating topic: I know of no studies which examine how different kinds of therapists operating with different conceptualisations of the body, of health, recovery and illness, *actually* succeed in working effectively together. This, surely, has to be a prime target for a future research agenda on issues of communication in alternative therapy.

My final theme returns to the issue with which the paper began – the impact of occupational interests on the flow of communication between different kinds of healers and their patients. Here, however, I want to pursue this argument from a different perspective – one which involves a brief excursion into a social constructionist view of scientific knowledge, and a contemporary example to show how these issues have been reflected in terms of recent practice.

For a long time in the history of sociological thought, sociologists were content, when they examined science at all, to leave the products of scientific work ('knowledge') outside their investigations. After all, it was argued, if scientific knowledge was determined by the unchanging nature of the physical world, it could have no social component (Merton 1973, Mannheim 1936).

Faith in this position was first undermined by philosophical work which showed that the idea of the growth of objective knowledge about the world by a process of 'conjecture and refutation' (Popper 1963) was ultimately unsustainable (e.g., Kuhn 1962, and especially Feyerabend 1975). Once the philosophers had broken the back of objectivist accounts of knowledge (i.e., that scientific findings were ultimately contingent on the nature of 'reality'), sociologists were not slow in making further advances against the traditional orthodoxy. Now, scientific knowledge was rather seen as a *socially constructed interpretation* of the natural world and its processes (e.g., Mulkay 1979).

How might this process work? If it is accepted that decisions about the acceptability of the results of scientific investigation are governed by sets of rules, then it is possible to see how a social component can readily intrude into the production of 'legitimate knowledge'. Rules, after all, always require application and interpretation. Two rules of particular importance as far as the reception of scientific results are concerned are the rules about criteria of *adequacy* (was the experimental work properly controlled and designed?); and *consistency* (are the results in line with established and accepted theory?).

It is quite clear that the scientific community – including that working within medicine – uses these rules in a *flexible* rather than in a consistent way. For example, the results of experimental work which fail to meet all criteria of adequacy may be accepted (for publication, for example) because the results are firmly consistent with accepted knowledge. Similarly, research which is inadequate and inconsistent may be published because it can subsequently be shown that orthodoxy is not threatened: drawing attention to experimental weaknesses will invalidate the findings.

However, results which are adequate but inconsistent pose a problem. Much can be at stake here. Received knowledge, with all its personal reputations, careers and employment generating research budgets, may be threatened by such work. In these circumstances, adequate but theory inconsistent findings may be undermined by asking the research team which produced them to meet new criteria of adequacy. This may involve showing that the results were *not* fraudulently produced (a rather difficult condition to meet!). Such a tactic seems to have been employed against Benveniste's work (Davenas et al 1988) on the activity of homoeopathic potencies – but this is not my main example, and I do not wish to pursue it further here.

Interestingly, Kleijnen et al's (1991) survey of 107 controlled and published trials of homoeopathy, which they reported in the *British Medical Journal*, lends support to the above theses: 84 of the trials failed to meet criteria of adequacy and 66 of these had produced results inconsistent with established physical and chemical theory (i.e., they had shown positive activity by homoeopathic potencies).

My main example, however, concerns the Bristol Cancer Help Centre (BCHC) in the UK. This had an international reputation for employing a variety of complementary and holistic techniques in its treatment programme. In 1986 it invited the medical establishment to assess the results of its work. The research team was led by Professor Tim McElwain; the project was to be supervised by the Institute of Cancer Research and was funded by two of the largest cancer charities, the Imperial Cancer Research Fund (ICRF) and the Cancer Research Campaign (CRC).

The research protocol was originally intended to cover two issues. Firstly, how did the survival rates of patients treated for breast cancer at Bristol compare with those receiving hospital treatment alone? Secondly, how did the quality of life of the Bristol group compare with that of the people being treated conventionally? The fieldwork was intended to last for at least five years.

What subsequently happened as the research developed had a profound impact on the women who were being treated at Bristol and on the reputation of complementary therapy in the UK. On the basis of only two years of fieldwork (June 1986 – June 1988), the research team chose to publish some preliminary results based on 334 women from the BCHC and 461 people receiving hospital treatment alone (Bagenal et al 1990). These results were leaked to the press a week beforehand, and featured prominently on the news programmes of all four major British television channels. Publication was accompanied by a major press conference in which Professor McElwain claimed that their work showed that women whose breast cancer had spread who chose to use complementary therapy were twice as likely to die compared to those choosing conventional treatment, and that metastasis free women who went to the BCHC after hospital treatment were three times more likely to relapse than patients who continued with regular therapy. In Professor McElwain's blunt words, Bristol women *"relapsed faster and died faster"* (Channel 4 1992).

According to Richard Smith, editor of the *British Medical Journal*, many medical representatives at the news conference greeted Professor McElwain's findings *"with glee"* (BBC 2 1995).

The research team, then, had apparently succeeded in confirming Professor

McElwain's previously enunciated views that complementary therapy was *"mumbo jumbo – we just can't do business with these people"* (BBC 2 1995).

The only problem with this was that Professor McElwain's team had done nothing of the sort. As people soon began to point out (including the BCHC which shortly afterwards organised a press conference in its own defence), the research failed to meet normal criteria of experimental adequacy, and so the preliminary results produced by the team should not have been taken seriously. In particular, the women who received hospital treatment only were badly matched with their Bristol counterparts; the research team had used less than half the number of controls as originally agreed in the research protocol; the Bristol women were more seriously ill than the women in the comparison group, and were younger so that the cancer would probably have spread more quickly; and while the raw data actually showed that they were three times *less* likely to relapse than the hospital patients, the complicated regression analysis used by the research team to analyse the data had successfully converted this risk to the *opposite* magnitude for publication purposes. Finally, the second aim of the original research protocol – the quality of life survey – had never actually been pursued by the McElwain team at all. Since the BCHC had never claimed to increase survival rates of cancer patients in the first place, but rather to add 'life to years', this was a serious omission.

It is difficult not to conclude that the particular research, occupational and career interests of the professional medical establishment and (here) its charitable sponsors had, in this case, interpreted the criteria of adequacy regarding the findings of the Bristol research programme in a particularly loose way, because the results apparently confirmed what was 'commonsensically' expected. The 'theory consistent' result *had* to be that complementary therapies were either innocuous or dangerous when compared to conventional cancer treatment, and this was what was 'found'. The *Lancet*, the journal which had carried the original report, was similarly culpable: the article had not undergone the normal process of statistical peer review. More sinisterly, it appears that Professor Karol Sikora, who had always been sceptical of the McElwain findings, had apprised the ICRF of this fact, and had intended to appear at the press conference which announced the original findings in order to add (with the support of the BCHC) some cautionary words. He never actually made it. According to BBC 2 (1995), he may well have come under pressure from the ICRF not to appear.

The stress of this incident was not all one way. The BCHC had felt besieged and threatened, but Professor McElwain himself, reportedly suffering from stress and overwork, sadly committed suicide some two weeks after the publication of his report. However, although the flaws in this work are now widely accepted, even by the charities which sponsored it, it has not been formally withdrawn, and the BCHC's reputation continues to suffer.

In sum, then, I have attempted to indicate some of the factors which, from a sociological point of view, can be seen to impinge on the process of communication about alternative therapy: occupational and status group interests; the postmodern condition itself and the problems of identity and the construction of 'the self' which it creates; incompatibilities among conceptualisations of the body, health and illness; and the propensity of research groups to engage in the selective interpretation of the rules by which knowledge claims are judged when powerful sectional interests are threatened.

There are clearly more avenues to explore. Poststructuralist thought, with its radical critique of knowledge and meaning, is a rather obvious candidate. But that must wait for a future paper.

References

Anderson, Jørgen Østergard
1995 "Lifestyles, Consumption and Alternative Therapies", paper delivered to *INRAT* internal seminar, March 20-22.

Bagenal, F. S. et al
1990 "Survival of Patients with Breast Cancer Attending Bristol Cancer Help Centre", in: *The Lancet,* 336: 606-10.

Barker, J. Ellis
1932 See his remarks in: *Heal Thyself,* June 1932: 221-4; July 1932: 267-8, 279, 290; and September 1932: 367, 371-2, 394-8.

BBC 2
1995 "Taking Liberties: The Cancer War Story", May 23.

Channel 4
1992 "Free For All: Cancer Positive", July 23.

Clarke, Graham
1994 "Homoeopathy and the New NHS", in: *Homoeopathy,* 44: 138-40. See especially p. 138.

Coulter, Harris L.
1973-7 *Divided Legacy: A History of the Schism in Medical Thought,* 3 vols., Wehawken Book Company: Washington.

Davenas, E. and Benveniste, J.
1988 "Human Basophil Degranulation Triggered by Very Dilute Antiserum Against IgE", in: *Nature,* 333: 816-8.

Feyerabend, Paul
1975 *Against Method,* New Left Books: London.

Giddens, Anthony
1991   *Modernity and Self Identity,* Polity Press: Cambridge.

Kleijnen, J. et al
1991   "Clinical Trials of Homoeopathy", in: *British Medical Journal,* 302: 316-23.

Kuhn, Thomas S.
1962   *The Structure of Scientific Revolutions,* University of Chicago Press: Chicago.

Lyotard, Jean-Francois
1984   *The Postmodern Condition,* Manchester University Press: Manchester.

Mannheim, Karl
1936   *Ideology and Utopia,* Routledge and Kegan Paul: London.

McGuire, Meredith
1995   "Alternative Therapies: The Meaning of Bodies in Knowledge and Practice", in: H. Johannessen, S. Gosvig Olesen and J. Østergard Andersen (eds.): *Studies in Alternative Therapy 2, Body and Nature,* pp. 15-32, Odense University Press: Odense.

Merton, Robert K.
1973   *The Sociology of Science,* University of Chicago Press: Chicago.

Mulkay, Michael
1979   *Science and the Sociology of Knowledge,* George Allen and Unwin: London.

Nicholls, Phillip A.
1988   *Homoeopathy and the Medical Profession,* Croom Helm: London.

Peterson, M. J.
1978   *The Medical Profession in Mid-Victorian London,* University of California Press: Berkeley.

Popper, Sir Karl
1963   *Conjectures and Refutations,* Routledge and Kegan Paul: London.

Rothstein, William G.
1972   *American Physicians in the Nineteenth Century: From Sects to Science,* Johns Hopkins University Press: Baltimore.

Society of Homoeopaths
1981-94 *Registers,* Northampton.

Spickard, James V.
1995   "Body, Nature and Culture in Spiritual Healing", in: H. Johannessen, S. Gosvig Olesen and J. Østergard Andersen (eds.): *Studies in Alternative Therapy 2, Body and Nature,* pp. 65-81, Odense University Press: Odense.

Weber, Max
1922   *Wirtschaft und Gesellschaft,* translated as *Economy and Society: An Outline of Interpretive Sociology* (by G. Roth and G. Wittich), Bedminster Press: New York, 1968.

Four Aspects of Placebo

– based on a review of the literature and a qualitative interview investigation among general practitioners and alternative therapists[1]

by Toke Barfod

The placebo concept plays a central role in discussions about alternative therapy, but it is, however, very ambiguous. This ambiguity can affect communication between different sorts of therapists, and may confuse scientists in their design and interpretation of placebo-controlled trials. This paper attempts to shed light on the complexity of the placebo concept by discussing four aspects:

Definitions – placebo and placebo effect
Empirical evidence – evidence for the healing potential of the placebo effect
Placebo as understood by therapists – preliminary report of interview study
Placebo in scientific trials – problems inherent in the methodology

Definitions

History of the placebo concept
The term "placebo" comes from Latin, meaning *"I shall please."* Its meaning today is not merely a translation from Latin. To understand the underlying meaning of the word, one must look at its historical development. Shapiro has studied the history of the placebo concept (Shapiro 1968), and his findings are summarised below.

The word "placebo" entered the English vocabulary in the 13th century, when a placebo meant: *"A song for the dead."* This meaning of the word arose from the fact that the first word in a ritual song at the Catholic funeral was "Placebo . . ."[2]

---

[1] This paper is based on diploma work done on a one-year research scholarship at the Institute of General Practice, University of Aarhus, with financial support from the Danish Medical Research Council, Fonden af 1870 and Nycomed DAK. The study was supervised by Dr. Jørgen Lous and Professor Uffe Juul Jensen. The author is a medical student in his final year. Part of the results were presented at "Médecine plurielle ou pluralité des médecines," 9-10 June 1995, Lausanne, and at the 9th Nordic Congress on General Practice, 19-22 June 1995, Uppsala. I thank Dr. Jørgen Lous, Dr. Flemming Bro, and John Anderson for help with the manuscript.

[2] The full first line of the song was: *"Placebo Domino in regione vivorum,"* meaning: *"I shall please the Lord in the land of the living"* or: *"I shall walk before the Lord in the land of the living"* (Shapiro 1968).

The professional mourners were also said to "sing placebo". These mourners were often looked down upon, and soon the word also took on a general, secular meaning: "A flatterer, sycophant, parasite." This meaning was kept for centuries. Much later, at the beginning of the 17th century, the word "placebo" entered the medical language and meant: *"Any medicine adapted more to please than benefit the patient."* It was not until the first half of the twentieth century that the placebo is described in a dictionary as inactive. In the late 1940s, the first placebo-controlled trials of pharmacological substances were performed. Since then, a "placebo" has been understood to be a kind of therapy as well as a device for control in trials.

Definition of placebo
According to Grünbaum (Grünbaum 1986), the word "placebo" is used in medical literature for: *"a treatment without specific effect."* A placebo is given in two different contexts: 1) in placebo-controlled *trials*, in which specific treatments are evaluated, and the placebo-treated control-group is used as a basis for comparison; 2) in practical *therapy*, in which the placebo is given to cure, help, satisfy or pacify the patient. In practical therapy, the placebo can be given either as a) the *"intentional"* placebo, when the therapist knows that he is giving a treatment without specific effect, or b) the *"inadvertent"* placebo, when the therapist believes that the treatment has a specific effect, though it has not.

The expression "a placebo" is used synonymously with "a placebo *treatment*." "Placebo *effect*" is seen as distinct from a placebo, because the placebo effect is seen not only as the effect of placebos. It is also seen as something that may contribute to the effects of specific therapies.

Placebo effect
The term "placebo effect" is used in at least three different ways:
1) Some use the term placebo effect synonymously with the effects of beliefs (Hahn 1985). The benefit of this definition is that it is specific. The definition does not include all the other effects of a therapy that are not "specific." And this may be of benefit in relation to practical therapy, in which many "unspecific" factors are important parts of the therapeutic situation, and there might be a reluctance to sum up their effects as "just a placebo effect".

2) Others use the term "placebo effect" covering the sum of reasons for improvement or cure in a placebo-treated control group (Bergin 1994, Ernst 1995). In other words, the term "placebo effect" may cover the reasons for cure *after* a treatment with a placebo. This definition includes the *perceived* effects of spontaneous fluctuations in disease and symptom remission, and

the perceived effects of regression towards the mean caused by measurement imprecision. Furthermore, this understanding of placebo effect also includes the *possible* healing effects of the history-taking and diagnosis, the effect of the placebo treatment itself, and the effects of being in a trial (often called Hawthorne-effect) (Ernst 1995).
In relation to placebo-controlled trials it seems relevant to use "placebo effect" in this way as a common term covering the reasons for cure in the placebo-treated control group. In this situation, the "placebo effect" is used as a term for the effects of all the factors that are of no interest in the particular experiment.

3) Others define the placebo effect as the difference in outcome between a placebo-treated group and an untreated control group (Ernst 1995, Gøtzsche 1994).
This equals the effects *caused* by the placebo treatment itself. This definition is sensible if there is interest in the effect of the "unspecific" parts of therapy. It is a definition that is currently advised in prestigious medical journals (Ernst 1995, Gøtzsche 1994). However, experiments seldom include an untreated control group as well as a placebo-treated control group (Ernst 1995). As we shall see later, the definition is not without complications. It has recently been concluded that *"the placebo concept as presently used cannot be defined in a logically consistent way"* (Gøtzsche 1994).

Placebo effects are caused by incidental factors
In standard terminology, the placebo is said to be *"a treatment without specific effect"* (Grünbaum 1986). It may, however, still have a "placebo effect." The placebo effect may, as we shall see, be just as "specific" in its consequences as the "specific effects." Thus, if we talk about the placebo effect as part of specific therapies (and not only as the effect of placebos), how are the specific and the placebo effects distinguishable from each other?

The specific effect and the placebo effect are separated, not by their *kind* of effects, but by the factors *causing* their effects. This becomes clear when we turn to the trials of clinical pharmacology, the context in which the concept of placebo as a control-treatment in trials was born.

In trials of pharmacological products, the "specific effects" can easily be defined as the effects of the pharmacological contents of the pills, and the "placebo effects" can be defined as the effects of the patients' psychological responses (Shapiro 1978). Imagine for example a situation in which the effect of a pill is disappearance of pain. If the pain stopped because of the pharmacological substance of the pill, then it is a specific effect. If it stopped because of the patient's psychological response to the taking of the pill, then it is a placebo effect.

In this way the separation of the placebo effect from the specific effect is made by equating "placebo effect" with "caused by a psychological response." However, this way of separating the two effects cannot be used directly in the description of other, more *complex* therapies, e.g., therapies that include elements of psychotherapy. Because if the effects were so separated, psychotherapy would be nothing but placebo. Therefore, Grünbaum explicated the definitions given above. He did so in an attempt to overcome the trouble that arises when we use the terminology of the scientific method of clinical pharmacology, i.e., the placebo-controlled clinical trial, in the description and investigation of more complex therapies.

Grünbaum suggested replacing the term "specific effects" with something less ambiguous (Grünbaum 1986). "The specific effect" could instead be called "the effect of the *defining* parts of the therapy."[3] According to Grünbaum, all forms of treatment consist of defining as well as incidental parts (or factors). The *defining* parts are the ones that constitute the therapy. Without them, it cannot be said to be such a therapy. The *incidental* parts of the therapy are ones that are normally present in the therapy, but do not have to be present for the therapy to be of the specified kind. As examples, the defining part of a therapy such as an operation for gallstones is the removal of gallstones. One incidental factor is the anaesthesia.

Thus, rephrasing Grünbaum, *placebo effects can be defined as the effects of the "incidental" parts of the treatment*, and *a placebo can be defined as a therapy that does not exert its effects through the "defining" parts of the treatment*.

There could be two reasons for the defining parts of a therapy not to have a healing effect. First, such defining factors may not be present in the therapy, e.g., for placebo tablets in trials (where the defining part of the therapy, the pharmacological substance, has deliberately been removed). Second, the defining factors of a therapy may not have a healing effect, e.g., some herbal medicines. Whether such placebos have healing potentials or not depends on the effect of their "incidental" factors, the placebo effect.

This definition of placebo fits well with the use of placebos in pharmacological trials, in which the therapy means the pharmacological substance. It also fits well with placebo-controlled trials of more complex therapies.

However, the definition does have a weakness. Namely, that the question

---

3 Grünbaum calls the "defining" factors "characteristic". However, since he explains thoroughly that these "characteristic" factors are the ones that define the therapy, they are here called "defining".

about whether a therapy is a placebo is determined by a relation between the definition of the therapy and reality. If the definition of the therapy correctly singles out the active elements in it as defining for the therapy, then the therapy is not a placebo. Nevertheless, if the definition of the therapy includes only parts of the therapy that are really unimportant to the outcome, then the treatment is a placebo. This means that his definition of placebo has been unable entirely to solve the problem of using the concept in describing complex therapies in which the therapy's defining parts are often less self-evident than in clinical pharmacology.

This can be illustrated by an example. Imagine, for instance, that it is an objectively stated fact that reflexology *does* lessen some sorts of headaches. It has also been shown that it works by way of massage, the relaxation and the contact between patient and therapist, but that the pressure on particular areas of the foot gives no extra effect. Then, *if* the relaxation and the contact are understood as defining parts of the therapy, without which it cannot be called reflexology, then their effects are not to be considered placebo effects. However, *if* reflexology is defined as pressure on specific areas, reflexology is a pure placebo-treatment. Thus, Grünbaum's explanation may be the most logically consistent, but it is not without complications.

Emperical Evidence

In an often cited article from 1955 by H. K. Beecher (Beecher 1955), it is claimed that one third of the patients get well because of placebo effect, and that this fraction is constant. This myth has survived, perhaps because it provides its proponents with an alibi not to pay further attention to the "unspecific effects" and the subtleties of therapy.

In Beecher's and many later reports of observed placebo effects, there have been no untreated control groups, so that spontaneous remission and regression towards the mean have not been controlled for. The results are therefore hard to interpret. However, other original reports of experiments with "placebo effects" supply us with information about the effects of "the unspecific healing factors" in therapy. My review of 45 original reports (Barfod 1995) led to the following conclusions:

- There is a substantial healing potential in the patient's motivation to get well, in the patient's belief in the treatment (even unconscious beliefs as conditioned responses), and in the expressed optimism and attention of the therapist.

- Some experiments show that there is a healing potential in the mere ingestion of tablets, but others show that the same effect can be achieved by communicating that no treatment is needed.

- These factors have mainly been investigated and shown to have an effect on pain, psychiatric disorders, patient satisfaction and illness behaviour, but also in more physical measurements such as blood pressure and size of inflammatory swelling.

- Possibly these factors cure or help about one third of the patients *on average*. The magnitude and duration of the effect differ considerably from trial to trial, from patient to patient, from disease to disease, and from therapist to therapist.

- The effects may be negative (nocebo) as well as positive.

- Mechanisms behind the effects of the *placebo-tablets alone* include: direct physiological responses such as the release of endorphins, responses stemming from a healthy behaviour modification in response to belief in the pill, and the effects of the symbolic functions of the tablet.

Thus, there is some healing potential in these different aspects of therapy, a potential that produces the so-called placebo effect. However, the realisation and use of this potential are very inconstant.

Placebo as Understood by Therapists

Background
This paper has already discussed the difficulties of defining "placebo" and "placebo effect," and it has summarised the proof of the healing potentials of placebo effects. To find out how therapists act, think and feel about placebo in practice, the medical literature was searched for empirical studies on the subject. Six questionnaire-surveys (Goodwin 1979, Goldberg 1979, Gray 1981, Hofling 1955, Thomson 1982, Shapiro 1973) (please note that the most recent is from 1982), and two interview investigations were found (Meyer 1989, Andersen 1994). The studies investigated doctors and nurses. The findings are quite consistent, and it can be concluded that:

- Doctors and nurses are defensive about placebos. They are inclined to believe that others use placebos more often than they do themselves (Hofling 1955,

Thomson 1982). They are also inclined to define placebo so that their own kind of treatment is excluded from the definition (Shapiro 1973). One investigation found that the doctors and nurses often talk about placebo with inhibition (Meyer 1989).

- Placebos are used by most therapists, but most of them do it very seldom (Gray 1981, Goodwin 1979).

- Placebos are mainly used to treat pain in demanding and troublesome patients, usually with good effect (Gray 1981, Goodwin 1979, Goldberg 1979).

- When a patient gets well on a placebo treatment, the therapist often interprets this proof of psychological origins of the complaints[4] (Gray 1981, Goodwin 1979).

- General practitioners differ from other doctors by including pharmacologically active drugs more often in their definition of placebo (Shapiro 1973).

These studies were mainly concerned with the use of "pure placebos" such as tablets of calcium or injections of water. Only limited attention was given to therapists' thoughts about placebo *effects* unrelated to placebo-treatment, and no study was found relating to alternative therapists' thoughts about placebo.

Aim
The aim of this part of the study was to explore the ways in which some general practitioners (GPs) and alternative therapists (ATs) in Denmark today think about placebo treatment and placebo effects. For example, what do they mean by the words *placebo* and *placebo effect*? Do they consider that the placebo effect is an important part of their therapy? What are their attitudes to the use of placebos and placebo effects? The aim was also to investigate whether their thoughts about placebo were related to their attitudes to "the other group of therapists," i.e., GPs' and ATs' attitudes toward each other.

Methods and material
A qualitative interview investigation was applied, inspired by Strauss and Corbin's description of "grounded theory" (Strauss 1990) and by the phenomen-

---

[4] This is a dangerous mistake, because the patients may thereby be deprived of effective somatic treatment (Goodwin 1979)(Goldberg 1979).

ological method of Giorgi (Giorgi 1994). Eight GPs and seven ATs from Århus and the surrounding countryside were selectively sampled. Whenever possible, the sampling of ATs was restricted to those trained and formally organised according to their profession, receiving payment for their services. The most frequently used methods of alternative therapy (Launsø 1994) were represented (reflexology, acupuncture, spiritual healing, homeopathy and herbal medicine).

Apart from these restrictions, the people interviewed (the informants) were selected for maximum variation with respect to factors related to their placebo concept (e.g., education, speciality, age, gender, types of patient, attitude toward other group of therapists). This was done in an attempt to cover the "causal field" and obtain qualitative representativeness of the data (Sandelowski 1986; Wackerhausen 1991).

As a custom (Strauss 1990), the sampling and the analysis were done alternately and in tandem. The informants were interviewed individually. These interviews, tape-recorded and transcribed by the researcher, each lasted for about one hour.

In the analysis, the text was fragmented and grouped into themes. The thematic fragments were further subcategorised, and patterns of relations between subcategories from different themes were sought.

Data of	GPs	ATs
Age, approx.	40 – 60 years	40 – 70 years
Sex	5 male, 3 female	1 male, 6 female
Years of experience	1 – 35 years	3 months – 25 years
Clients	Various	Various
Time with each pt.	Usually 15 minutes	Usually 1 hour
Special interests	Various specialities	As mentioned above
Scientific work	Not at all – very little – some	Not at all – very little
Religion, roughly:	Various (Christian or atheists)	Various (private religions)

Preconceptions
It is useful in qualitative research to counteract the inevitable effects of the preconceptions of the researcher by trying to explain them in advance (Malterud 1993). My conscious preconceptions about GPs, ATs and placebo before starting the study, may be summarised as follows:

I expected the individual GPs to hold contradictory views about placebo concepts. I had only vague ideas about the placebo concepts of the ATs – I thought that perhaps some would not even know the word. My personal view was that the "incidental parts" of most alternative therapies were responsible for a great deal of their healing potentials, but that beliefs were not necessarily the main factor among these.

I realised during the study that from its start, I had fostered a critical attitude towards the paternalistic way by which GPs try to achieve placebo effects. However, I changed this attitude as the study progressed.

Preliminary findings
Very different placebo concepts and attitudes towards the use of placebo effects were found. Some of them will be presented below as brief quotes.

There were interesting connections between subcategories. The GP's views on placebo seemed to differ according to their attitude towards alternative therapy. Interestingly, the AT's views on placebo seemed to differ according to their degree of education. Citations below are therefore grouped according to these subcategories. The GPs are labelled "conventional" if they did not offer alternative therapies themselves, and "alternative" if they treated some of their patients with an alternative therapy. They are labelled "alternative-critical" and "alternative-positive" according to their attitudes. The ATs are labelled "academic" if they had some sort of education from the university (usually not related to their therapy), otherwise "nonacademic".

The presented citations are edited and not word-to-word transcriptions. When they express the viewpoints of more than one informant, the precise number of informants is not given, because in qualitative research the selective sampling makes such numbers irrelevant. The findings are presented under three headings:

1) The way they talked about placebo effects
2) Attempts to enhance placebo effects
3) "The other group of therapists" and placebo

1) The way they talked about placebo effects
The conventional GPs often talked about the placebo effect as: *"Something that can be used for therapeutic reasons."* An alternative-critical GP talked about the placebo effect as: *"The effect of ineffective therapies."* Alternative-positive GPs often talked about placebo effects as: *"A part of every treatment."*

The nonacademic ATs and the alternative GPs usually talked differently about placebo effects. Some said: *"It is a concept only relevant in trials."* Like one conventional doctor above: *"It is the effect of ineffective therapies."* Others: *"There is no placebo effect at all in my therapy,"* but admitted that there was a placebo effect in a method that was used earlier or in other alternative therapies. Some emphasised that the placebo effect was: *"Uncontrollable, and the same in all therapies."* By contrast with the others in this group, one alternative GP was very enthusiastic about using placebo effects: *"It is an important part of most treatments, and you should always try to 'sell' the treatment as well as possible. But only when there is no doubt that the particular treatment is needed, of course."*

Several academic ATs had a very broad conception of the placebo effect. They included: *"All mind-body-interactions"* in their definition of placebo effect. All the academic ATs regarded such interactions as the main part of their treatment.

2) Attempts to enhance placebo effects

Several conventional GPs said something like: *"On rare occasions I feel constrained to prescribe some medicine, even though I don't think the patient needs any pharmacological substance. I prescribe it to some patients who really believe in and want some medicine. First, I try to convince them that no medicine is needed. But sometimes I do not succeed in this, because it is not possible to change everybody. Then, I prescribe some harmless medicine with only weak pharmacological potentials, as for instance vitamin B or pain killers."*

The older GPs tended to use paternalistic or manipulating ways of achieving placebo effects, e.g., by explaining the benefits of a medicine more thoroughly than its drawbacks. The younger GPs focused more on trying to achieve placebo effects through honest and thorough explanations. One newly established GP said: *"The placebo effect of paternalism has great healing potentials. But I can't use it, I'm too young."* Last, no GP claimed use of "pure placebo" without any pharmacological substance, such as tablets of calcium.

The ATs also focused on: *"Honesty and information."* As mentioned, most did not perceive placebo effects as a manipulable part of their therapy. Some even *"deliberately avoid to consider the placebo effect,"* either because it was generally considered *"impossible to find out about placebo effects,"* or because the placebo effect was perceived as *"depending on fine things,"* that for moral reasons should be left to themselves. One AT used calcium tablets as placebo, while telling the patient that he was receiving a medicine. The AT did so not to achieve healing placebo effects, but: *"To calm the patient, while waiting for the real medicine to work."* Another AT said that it was a main part of her therapy: *"To convince the patient that it is crucial to think positively."* Others talked about: *"Using the healing power of a wish to benefit the patient."* One of these talked about this effect as: *"A healing in disguise."* She used this power secretly while she was doing the "regular" therapy, because she did not want to upset the patient by saying that she was also performing healing. She strongly connected this healing power with meditation and prayer.

3) "The other group of therapists" and placebo
The alternative-positive GPs said about ATs and placebo: *"The patients have more faith in the alternative therapists, and therefore the alternative therapists have more placebo effect,"* or: *"The alternative therapists are generally more charismatic than the doctors, because if they were not, many of them would not get any patients. And therefore they have more placebo effect than many doctors."* One thought: *"Often the alternative therapists know more about psychosomatics than doctors,"* and some said: *"It is good when the patient believes in an alternative therapist, because you should never take away the patient's hope."*

A more alternative-critical GP said: *"The placebo effect cannot cure anyone,"* while another remarked: *"The placebo effects of the alternative therapists seem to be short-lasting."* However, this GP still found placebo effects important in his own therapy.

Several ATs said: *"The doctors have more placebo effects than the alternative therapists, because the patients believe more in them."* Other, more critical ATs meant: *"The doctors are often not very good at handling patients, and therefore have very little positive placebo effect."*

Discussion of findings and validity in interview study
The presentation of the results is meant to give a broad picture of the ways in which these GPs and ATs think about placebo. A few points may, however, be pointed out and discussed.

First, the meaning of the term placebo effect differed very much within both groups. Thus, the pluralism of placebo concepts was as big as in the literature. Second, several conventional GPs understood the placebo effect as part of their therapy. Most of them tried to maximize the placebo effect for the benefit of their patients. The ATs who had some academic education perceived the placebo effect as a very important part of their therapy. So the defensiveness found in earlier studies of the attitudes of doctors and nurses could not be found among the GPs, and certainly not among the ATs with academic education. Third, the ATs without academic education, and most of the alternative doctors, did not talk about placebo effects as a manipulable part of their therapy. They said that it was a concept only relevant to research, or that there was no placebo effect in their therapy, that the placebo effect was not to be manipulated, or that it was the same in all therapies.

The reasons for these differences in attitude are probably the combined effects of differences in cosmology, semantics and degree of defensiveness towards this medically defined term.

The *internal validity* of this study, i.e., the validity of *qualitative content* of the presented statements and the *relations* between subcategories, should be ensured by the methods used (i.e., what was meant, by which group, and the patterns of meaning, in this sample).

Other members of the two groups of therapists, and not only the interviewed sample, are likely to hold views on placebo that are similar to the ones presented. Therefore, the description of the *qualitative contents* of meanings can be generalized as well. However, the extent by which the *relations* between subcategories can be generalized cannot be ensured in this kind of study (e.g., what group of therapists meant what). The extent by which the relations between subcategories can be generalized can only be viewed as a likely hypothesis.

Placebo in Scientific Trials

The placebo-controlled trial remains a very strong method of investigation. However, some general problems in placebo-controlled trials are probably more profound in the investigation of alternative therapies than in the investigation of most conventional medical therapies. Four such problems will be mentioned here.

Ethics

There are ethical problems in giving placebos to patients in trials, if this means that the patients are deprived of known active therapy (Rothman 1994). This is often a problem in the evaluation of alternative therapies, because the therapists often believe so strongly in the effect of their therapies that they find it unethical to perform placebo-controlled trials.

Visible elements

When the presence or the absence of the active elements of the therapy is easily detectable by the patient or the therapist, it becomes difficult to obtain double-blinding (Greenberg 1994). However, it may also be worthwhile to compare the general effect of therapies without double-blinding them. After all, if there is a healing effect of the patient's and the therapist's beliefs about the therapeutic potentials of the treatment, then could this effect not be seen as a valid part of the therapy, which should not necessarily be controlled for?

Complex therapies

It is difficult to design placebos for the evaluation of "complex" therapies. As I have already discussed, the definition of a placebo as *a treatment that does not exert its effects through the defining parts of the therapy*, points to the importance of the way in which the therapy is defined. In complex therapies, e.g., reflexology, where the healing potential of many interacting factors is often acknowledged, it can be difficult to point out the "defining factors". To assess the relative importance of the different parts of a complex therapy, *"component control trials"* may be used instead of placebo-controlled trials (Borkovec 1985). In component control trials, the factors whose relative importance one wishes to investigate are omitted from the control treatment. This control treatment is, however, not called a placebo, since its other active factors are also appreciated. However, also in placebo-controlled trials, the "incidental" factors of a therapy are usually present in the placebo treatment as well as in the specific treatment. Nevertheless, in placebo controlled trials the effects of these "incidental" factors are called a placebo effect and dismissed. Therefore, if the "incidental" factors are really an active part of the therapy, the healing potential of the therapy will be underestimated if the therapy is only investigated by placebo-controlled trials.

Fragile therapies and placebo-controlled trials
In placebo-controlled trials, the healing effect of beliefs and knowing is dismissed (Sullivan 1993). There are probably some therapies that lose much of their effectiveness when the patient and the therapist do not know whether the patient is receiving the specific therapy under investigation or a placebo. Such therapies will be more vulnerable to the procedure of placebo-control than others. They could be termed *"fragile"*. The effects of fragile therapies will, thus, be underestimated when compared with less fragile therapies, if the effects of the two treatments are judged from placebo-controlled trials. Therefore, such therapies should also be assessed with less intervening methods.

In health services research, it is implicitly assumed that the maximum effect of a therapy (termed "efficacy") is achieved under experimental circumstances (Aday 1993). It is assumed that the effect of the therapy in daily practice (termed "effectiveness") is usually smaller than the effect achieved under experimental circumstances (Aday 1993). These assumptions are probably built on empirical grounds. Still, they might not always be right. The experimental circumstances may be damaging to some therapies, even when no placebo is used as control. Because apart from being sensitive to the uncertainty, whether a "specific" treatment is given, some fragile therapies may also be weakened by other circumstances of scientific trials. Their effect may, for example, be diminished by the influence of the observer, by the experimental context, by the process of randomisation or by the double-blinding procedure. However, this last point about the effects of the experimental circumstances is not necessarily related to the problem of placebo in trials. It is related to the inherent bias of randomised, double-blind trials. It is therefore beyond the scope of this paper.

Conclusion

The concept of placebo plays a central role in many discussions about alternative therapy. However, many different definitions of the words "placebo" and "placebo effects" coexist in the literature. A placebo may be understood as a treatment that does not exert its effects through its defining parts. But perhaps the placebo concept as presently used cannot be defined in a sensible way. Therefore, it is often a good idea to replace the words "placebo" and "placebo effect" by more specific terms. When the words "placebo" and "placebo effect" are used, it is advisable to explain, what is meant by them or at least be conscious of their ambiguity.

There is empirical evidence for the healing potentials of the "nonspecific" or "incidental" parts of therapy. Their effects are often summed up under the term "placebo effect". By that they are made more mysterious than they need to be, and they become harder to investigate and manipulate. However, we should not let the ambiguity of the placebo concept lead us to neglect or look down on the potentials of these important parts of therapies.

Very different attitudes towards placebo effects exist among therapists. Though great variations in attitudes occur within the investigated groups of therapists, there are certain tendencies: It seems that "conventional" general practitioners (GPs) often perceive the placebo effect as a manipulable part of their therapy, whereas alternative therapists (ATs) without academic education, and "alternative" GPs do not, and that the ATs with some academic education perceive the placebo effect as perhaps the most important part of their therapy. These differences in language and attitude might disturb communication and understanding between GPs and ATs.

The ambiguity of the placebo concept might disturb our design and interpretation of placebo-controlled trials. Other possible biases inherent in the nature of placebo-controlled trials should also be considered when treatments are evaluated and compared. If the results of placebo-controlled trials are interpreted with these biases in mind, such trials remain one of our strongest tools for evaluation of therapies. Still, the many other ways of achieving scientific weight and accuracy in the evaluation of therapies should also be considered.

References

Aday, L. A., Begley, C. E., Lairson, D. R. and Slater, C. H.
1993   "Effectiveness, Concepts and Methods", in: *Evaluating the Medical Care System*, pp. 23-47, Health Administration Press: Ann Arbor, Michigan.

Andersen, L. O.
1994   *Placebo – Nocebo,* [Folklore dissertation], Københavns Universitet, (unpublished).

Barfod, T.
1995   *Placebo i Videnskab og Behandling* [diplomopgave] (Placebo in Science and Therapy [diploma work]), Institute of General Practice, University of Aarhus: Århus.

Beecher, H. K.
1955   "The powerful placebo", in: *JAMA*, 159: 1602-1606.

Bergin, A. E.
1994   *Handbook of Psychotherapy and Behaviour Change*, p. 744, John Whiley & Sons, Inc.: New York.

Borkovec, T. D.
1985   "Placebo: Defining the Unknown", in: L. White, B. Tursky and G. E. Schwartz (eds.): *Placebo: Theory, Research and mechanisms*, pp. 59-64, The Guilford Press: New York.

Ernst, E. and Resch, K. L.
1995   "Concept of true and perceived placebo effects", in: *British Medical Journal*, 311: 551-553.

Giorgi, A.
1994   "An Application of Phenomenological Method in Psychology", in: A. Giorgi, et al (eds.): *Duquesne Studies in Phenomenological Psychology*, pp. 82-103, Duquesne University: Pittsburg.

Goldberg, R. J., Leigh, H. and Quinlan, D.
1979   "The current status of placebo in hospital practice", in: *General Hospital Psychiatry*, 1: 196-201.

Goodwin, J. S., Goodwin, J. M. and Vogel, A. V.
1979   "Knowledge and use of placebos by house officers and nurses", in: *Ann. Intern. Med.*, 91: 106-110.

Gray, G. and Flynn, P.
1981   "A survey of placebo use in a general hospital", in: *General Hospital Psychiatry*, 3: 199-203.

Greenberg, R. P. and Fisher, S.
1994   "Suspended judgment – seeing through the double-masked design: a commentary", in: *Controlled Clinical Trials*, 15: 244-246.

Grünbaum, A.
1986   "The placebo concept in medicine and psychiatry", in: *Psychol. Med.*, 16: 19-38.

Gøtzsche, P. C.
1994   "Is there logic in the placebo?" in: *Lancet*, 344: 925-926.

Hahn, R. A.
1985 "A Sociocultural Model of Illness and Healing", in: L. White, B. Tursky, and G. E. Schwartz (eds.): *Placebo: Theory, Research and Mechanisms*, pp. 167-195, The Guilford Press: New York.

Hofling, C. K.
1955 "The place of placebos in medical practice", in: *G.P.*, 11: 103-107.

Launsø, L. and Brendstrup, E.
1994 "Forskning i Alternativ Behandling i Danmark" (Research in Alternative Therapy in Denmark), Sundhedsstyrelsens Råd vedrørende Alternativ Behandling i Danmark: Copenhagen.

Malterud, K.
1993 "Shared understanding of the qualitative research process. Guidelines for the medical researcher", in: *Family Practice*, 10: 201-206.

Meyer, U. A. and Kindli, R.
1989 "Plazebos und nozebos", in: *Ther. Umsch.*, 46: 544-554.

Rothman, K. J. and Michels, K. B.
1994 "The continuing unethical use of placebo controls", in: *N. Engl. J. Med.*, 331: 394-398.

Sandelowski, M.
1986 "The problem of rigor in qualitative research", in: *Advances in Nursing Science*, 8: 27-37.

Shapiro, A. K.
1968 "Semantics of placebo", in: *Psychiatric Quarterly*, 42: 653-696.

Shapiro, A. K. and Morris, L.
1978 "The Placebo Effect in Medical and Psychological Therapies", in: S. Garfield, and A. Bergin (eds.): *Handbook of Psychotherapy and Behavior Change*, pp. 369-410, John Wiley & Sons: New York.

Shapiro, A. K. and Struening, E.
1973 "Defensiveness in the definition of placebo", in: *Compr. Psychiatry*, 14: 107-120.

Strauss, A. and Corbin, J.
1990 *Basics of Qualitative Research*, Sage Publications: Newbury Park.

Sullivan, M. D.
1993 "Placebo controls and epistemic control in orthodox medicine", in: *J. Med. Philos.*, 18: 213-231.

Thomson, R. J. and Buchanan, W. J.
1982 "Placebos and general practice: attitudes to, and the use of, the placebo effect", in: *New Zealand Medical Journal*, 95: 492-494.

Wackerhausen, S.
1991 "Udvælgelse af Personer i Kvalitative Undersøgelser" (Selection of Persons in Qualitative Investigations [working paper]), Institute of Philosophy, Aarhus University: Aarhus.

The Placebo: Mysterious Forces or Investigating Complexity?

by Robert Lafaille

Yet in spite of the patently useless
and quite often dangerous treatments
offered throughout medical history,
people seemed to get better
(Ornstein & Sobel 1987: 77).

Overview and Historical Background

Placebo is a Latin expression which means "I will please" or translated more freely "I will care for." There is some evidence that the word stems from an incorrect translation of a passage in the Bible.[1] "Placebo" first meant a title for the form of certain Roman Catholic vespers for the dead. Later, its meaning changes to "flattery," "courtesan," and other similar words expressing the gaiety of post-Renaissance European court life (Jospe 1978: XIII). A definition of placebo as "a commonplace method or medicine" appeared in the 1787 edition of Quincy's Lexicon. In the 1811 edition of Harper's Medical Dictionary the word placebo was defined as *"an epithet given to any medium adopted more to please than to benefit the patient."* This definition has carried through to the twentieth century with recent revisions (Sanford 1994: 247). The concept of placebo became especially relevant when pharmacological investigations proved that pretended drugs (for example a similar capsule filled with sugar instead of the active component) affected the patient as the drug which the researcher expected would cure the illness or would have a certain therapeutical effect. Such a pretended medicament was called a placebo. The effect of it on the patient a placebo-effect. In contemporary medicine, the term placebo is not only used in the

---

[1] According to my information the verse "Placebo Domino . . ." (I shall please the Lord) is a Latin translation of Eusebius of verse 6 of Chapter 150 of the Psalmbook. The original Hebrew text would mean "I shall walk before the Lord . . .". But other sources refer to Psalm 114 of the Vulgate (Jospe 1978: XII) or to Psalm 166 verse 9 (Shapiro 1971: 440).

context of the pharmacological effectiveness of medicaments, but it has been extended to all forms of medical treatment which causes a circumscribed effect without the availability of a sufficient scientific concept or theory which could explain the caused effect.

Placebo is commonly defined by the well-known definition of Shapiro: *"A placebo is every therapeutical procedure (or one of its components) which is given freely to attain a certain effect, or directly causes an effect on symptoms, syndrome or illness, but which has no specific activity on the condition under treatment"* (Shapiro 1963) and *"A placebo is any therapy (or component of therapy) that is deliberately or knowingly used for its nonspecific, psychological, or psychophysiological effect, or that is used unknowingly for its presumed or believed effect on a patient, symptom, or illness, but which, unknown to patient and therapist, is without specific activity for the condition being treated"* (Shapiro 1971). Jospe (1978: XIV) proposed to substitute in the definition of Shapiro (1963) the phrase *"any therapeutic procedure ... which is without specific activity for a condition to be treated"* by *"that portion of the behavioral change that can be attributed to any therapeutic procedure that is without specific activity for the condition to be treated, as contrasted to the behavioral change due to mere passage of time, repeated testing, or other "spontaneous" influences occurring while on placebo"* (Jospe 1978: XIV).

What is a placebo and how does it function? The best way to explain this is by a classical experiment which was performed on medical students in a pharmacology class.

> "The professor lectured about stimulant and sedative medication, describing in detail the effects each has on the body and the side effects which might be anticipated with each. The students took either a pink pill, "the stimulant," or a blue pill, "the depressant," and recorded each other's symptoms, blood pressure, and heart rate. About half the students experienced specific anal measurable physiological reactions such as decreased blood pressure and heart rate as well as dizziness, watery eyes, abdominal pain, and the like. All the symptoms were consistent with the drug taken, either the stimulant or the depressant. But of course the students were given inert pills, whose color, coupled with the students' expectations, produced the effects" (Ornstein & Sorbel 1987: 79-80).

The role played by the placebo in contemporary medical practice as well as in medical history cannot be overlooked. The intelligent therapeutic use of placebos remains as much an issue today as it was centuries ago. Current medical literature indicates that reactions to placebos may involve practically any organ system in the body. Placebos are known to cause undesirable side effects.[2] Response to the administration of placebos tends to be varied and broad in extent throughout the population. To date, no single accepted explanation of the placebo effect has been advanced (Sanford 1994: 248). Cousins (1977) has summarised a variety of cases reported in the medical literature over 25 years that point toward the efficacy of various placebos. Both the extent and variety of the placebo effect are so great that it has been remarked that a study showing no response to a placebo might be suspected of lack of objectivity on that ground alone (Brodeur 1965).

In the literature a series of classical distinctions appears, which I will mention here. A distinction is made between a placebo that consists of an inactive substance (*inert* placebo) and an active (*non-inert* placebo). Besides one distinguishes an *exact* placebo as one that mimics all the physical characteristics of the experimental substance or treatment (Jospe 1978: XIII).

In pharmacological research, *drug response* (the behavioral change of subjects on drugs) is distinguished from *drug effect* (that portion of the behavioral change that can be attributed to the pharmacodynamic action of the drug). Analogously we can make a distinction between *placebo response* and *placebo effect*. According to Fisher the term placebo response refers to *"the behavioral change of subjects receiving placebo,"* whereas the term placebo effect means *"that portion of the behavioral change which can be attributed to the symbolic transaction of being given medication, as contrasted with the behavioral change due to mere passage of time, repeated testing or other 'spontaneous' influences occurring while on placebo"* (Jospe 1978: XIII). This means that one also has to make a distinction between giving a placebo and the placebo effects of this themselves!

Fisher (1970) distinguishes between placebogenic and prognostigenic variables. Placebogenic variables are nonspecific variables that contribute directly to placebo effects. Prognostigenic variables are nonspecific variables associated with spontaneous change over time; drug-placebo comparisons will be minimizing the more favourable the prognostic level.

A placebo can have various effects. Classical is to distinguish between a pos-

---

[2] Buncher (1972) points out that *"side effects from placebo therapy are even more extensive than the list of conditions that are aided by placebo. Headaches, nausea, vomiting, dizziness, diarrhea, pain, dermatitis, drowsiness, anxiety-nervousness, weakness-fatigue, dry mouth, abdominal pain, insomnia, urinary frequency, urticaria, loss of libido, tinnitus, and so forth, have all been caused by the administration of placebos"* (Sanford 1994: 250). Not all the results of placebos are positive and therapeutic. An entire range of symptoms including palpitations, drowsiness and headaches as well as diarrhea and nausea can be produced by placebos (Ornstein & Sobel 1987: 79).

itive and a negative placebo effect. A placebo that causes negative effects is called a *nocebo* (term proposed by Kissel and Barrucand 1964)(Jospe 1978: XIV). Various procedures were developed to discover placebo effects (Jospe 1978: XIII): 1) A *single-blind procedure* is one in which the patient does not know whether s/he is receiving an experimental or control substance (usually an inert placebo); 2) a *double-blind procedure* is one in which neither the patient nor physician (or others treating or evaluating) knows to which group patients have been assigned; 3) a *triple-blind procedure* is one where a preliminary study with placebos is carried out, after which the placebo reactors are excluded for the definitive study that follows. This procedure is questionable: it supposes that a "placebo personality" exists. Moreover a selection of persons is induced, from which one does not know the precise underlying mechanism. Regression artifacts as well as similar phenomena can then appear (see below).

Placebo in the Pharmacological Context

The situation in a pharmacological context is clear. The doctor or pharmacologist has a theoretical frame of reference about the effect and influence of medicines and a specific theory (hypothesis) about the effectiveness of the specific drug he is applying. When new effects are generated which cannot be explained by the pharmacological frame of reference, this effect is called a placebo-effect. To this one refers when speaking of *aspecific* effects of drugs (definition of Shapiro, see before).

The following mechanisms are described as possible explanations for the placebo effect in a pharmaceutical context (Placebo's ... 1975): 1) The effect of a drug (placebo) which through conditioned intake rituals exerts a certain influence, although it cannot have from a pharmacological point of view a single effect upon the complaint or symptom; 2) The effect of suggestive influence by other persons (physician, nurse, family), including the effect of having delivered a prescription by a doctor or the reception of drugs in a pharmacy; 3) The effect of a positive expectation because an identical looking drug appeared effective in the past; or the reverse, a negative expectation because a similar looking drug seemed to be ineffective (this is a special case of self-fulfilling prophecy).

In technical terms, the placebo effect can be represented as follows:

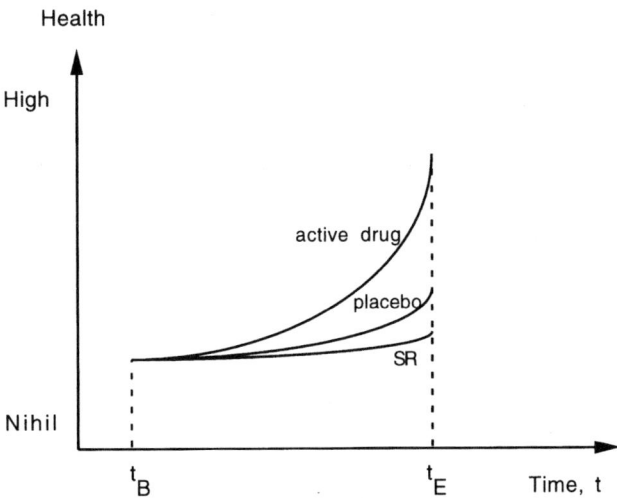

Figure 1: Differential effects of the active drug, placebo, and spontaneous remission

The real effect of a medicament is then the difference between the effect of the active drug (AD) and the placebo (P).[3] More exactly, it is the difference in surface between the two effect curves.

$$\text{Real effect AD} = \int_{B}^{E} f_{AD}(t)d(t) - \int_{B}^{E} f_{P}(t)d(t)$$

[1][4]

We can write this even more exactly by following an idea developed by Mabeck (1994). We can say that the observed effect of an active drug is the sum of the real, pure effect of the drug, the difference between its placebo and nocebo effects, the effect of spontaneous self-healing (spontaneous remission) and a random error term. In formula:

---

3   Mere differences are vulnerable for regression artifacts (see elsewhere in the text), because they do not rule them out. Better, although not perfect measures, are differences between values given by regression equations, because their partial regression coefficients control for all other observed variables.

4   B = Begin; E = End. Determining the endpoint is a theoretical matter, which implies a lot of methodological considerations (e.g., should the end point be the end of treatment or a point in time after the treatment has stopped, like for example a two-year post treatment evaluation?). In Fig. 1 the curves are very smooth. In practice, this might be more complex. An easier, but less accurate way to determine the differences is the ratio $(f_{AD}(t_E)/ f_P(t_E))$ at point E. In the literature we also find the Index of Drug Efficiency as a measure to define the relative impact of a drug and a placebo (see Evans 1974 as found in Jospe 1978: 31). This measurement is quite similar to the ratio mentioned before.

Total observed effect of AD = real effect of AD + (its placebo effect – its nocebo effect) + spontaneous remission + random error (including measurement errors) [2]

The term "placebo" can be investigated and calculated when giving a control group a real, exact placebo. It has to be the true value of the placebo effect, which means that the effect of spontaneous remission (SR) has to be subtracted. Spontaneous remission can be measured by observing a control group which is given no treatment at all.

Combining [1] and [2] it follows that in case there are no interactions between terms (warning: this has to be empirically proven, because in principle there are some possibilities for interactions, see below):

$$\int_B^E f_{AD}(t)d(t) = \text{Real effect of AD} + \int_B^E f_P(t)dt + \int_B^E f_{SR}(t)d(t) + \varepsilon$$

[3]

It has to be clear that

$$\int_B^E f_P(t)dt$$

is an observed value and as such is the result of positive and negative influences. We do not need to measure them separately.

In pharmacology this kind of view on placebo-effects might be useful. Placebo there is treated as a kind of special bias, and one is interested in the "true value" of the influence of the drug (research as bias free as possible). Placebos can mimic many effects usually thought to be the exclusive property of active pharmacological agents. Some of these are: a *time-effect curve* (a peak or maximum effect), a *cumulative effect* (increasing therapeutic effect with repeated doses), *carry-over effects* (persistence of effect after cessation of treatment), and an *inverse relationship* between efficacy of a placebo and the severity of a symptom (a more severe symptom responds less effectively) (Lasagna, Laties and Dohan 1958, Jospe 1978: XV). Some patients might even become addicted to placebos and will show many formal traits of drug dependence, including a tendency to increase the presumed dose, an inability to stop taking the placebos without psychiatric help, an almost compulsive desire to take the placebos, and withdrawal or abstinence syndrome on sudden deprivation of the "medication" (Vinar 1969, Jospe 1978: XV).

Transplantation of the Notion of Placebo to other Contexts

First, the term placebo is used in a variety of the literature in complementary medicine. There, the term is very often used in an aspecific way, referring to every result of alternative therapy that cannot be explained by classical medicine (see for an overview Van Dijk 1979, Fulder 1987). In this literature the notion of placebo often functions as a kind of ultimate and "mysterious" mechanism that serves as a sufficient explanation. It will also be clear that various professional groups use the placebo-effect as a kind of scientific legitimation for their professional interests. I think this kind of enlargement of the concept of placebo, although it serves certain (positive?) social functions, is undesirable in science.

Secondly, with the growing contribution of the human sciences in medicine, the concept of placebo is also quite often applied in these sciences. A transformation of context then appears: from pharmacology to human sciences. Such a transformation is not a noncommittal matter and scientists should reflect more deeply on its consequences. I think the human sciences have to investigate just these factors that are beyond the scope of the pharmacological frame of reference (see before). Therefore, the human sciences have to develop theoretical models to explain certain (treatment) effects. The placebo concept is of little use in these models. It can lead by a back door to declare relationships "mysterious" instead of gaining insight into complex treatment situations. Therefore, the placebo concept seems to me very inappropriate as a theoretical notion for the human sciences. Their task is just to help to reveal the unknown mechanisms in pharmacological research. So far, one has elaborated this line of thought too little.

Major Traps

Before discussing the mechanisms that could explain the workings of a placebo, it is necessary to mention some major traps. There are some phenomena that erroneously could be taken as placebo effects. In these cases it is either out of the question that one can speak of an effect, or the observed changes are not the effect of giving the placebo. Too little attention is given to these kinds of phenomena. To develop a sound methodology of placebo research, it is necessary to be aware of these topics.

First, I discuss the possibility of "regression to the mean." In case of regression to the mean the data show positive changes in health status, but these changes are not caused by any kind of treatment or drug, but by a certain kind of random phenomenon. How regression to the mean works, can best be explained by the *Board of Galton* (Dessens and Jansen 1982). This is a board with boxes above which a funnel is placed, which can contain balls that fall down on the board.

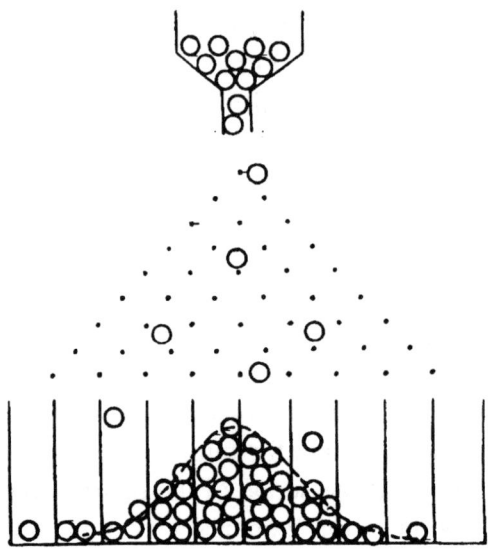

Figure 2: Board of Galton (borrowed from Dessens and Jansen 1982)

If the system functions well, the balls have to be distributed in the boxes according to a normal distribution. If now in a second stage – a second measurement – the balls that fell into one of the extreme positioned boxes at the left or right side would be given a number and put again in the funnel, then the numbered balls would not fall in these extreme boxes again, but would be distributed over all boxes according to a random pattern. The "extreme" scoring balls tend to distribute around the mean: they *regress to the mean*.

Regression to the mean can thus be the effect of a certain selection of the treatment group. Random sampling is insufficient to avoid regression to the mean. If one works with patients, there will always be a certain non-random selection. The possibility of regression to the mean is then always potentially present. It is quite difficult to control regression to the mean, because one does not observe this phenomenon directly. Comparison of means and variances between treatment and control groups is classical procedure, but it is only practicable in situations where a "pure" regression artefact appears. Mixed situations are much more difficult to detect.

A second unrecognized possibility of false conclusions is statistical artifacts. Much more than generally is accepted, statistical artifacts might appear. They naturally might lead to a conclusion that a placebo causes improvement in health, but there is no question of effect at all, because these positive data are created by the analytical tool used.

New insights, especially in chaos theory, showed that causal inference is much more complicated, than thought of in more classical methodologies. Cross-sectional analysis after all, might show random distributions (no causal relationships), although these data might be generated by "causal" chaotic mechanisms (Casti 1992). One has to be cautious here. Evidently many biochemical processes are chaotic of nature, but also human behavior contains much more chaotic behavior than is currently assumed (Van Geert 1991).

A third possibility, not to be confused with placebo effects, is the natural course of illnesses. Most illnesses are "self-limited." Even if one does nothing, most of the illnesses will be cured. So-called improvements are then not the result of the application of a placebo or a medicine, but of autonomous biological processes. A warning against psychological interpretations, which might overlook the natural course of illnesses, has to be given here, e.g., *"People are most likely to seek help at the worst point – if graphed, this would be the low point on the curve. Then, when they improve, they naturally attribute their improvement to the treatment they have received"* (Ornstein & Sobel 1987: 77). Obviously, regression artifacts wait in ambush.

It is also important to be aware that always (unknown) physiological ingredients might be active in a placebo. The application of a neutral substance like "sugar," "yeast" or some herbs, does not have to be so neutral. Especially the effect of herbs is still a highly unknown territory. A good example is the medieval practice of bloodletting (see also below). For a long time bloodletting was considered as a placebo effect. Modern chemical analyses would have shown that at least four specifically active biochemical substances are found in the leeches that counter different diseases (Ornstein & Sobel 1987: 77). Medical history offers many similar examples.

Explanations for the Placebo Effect

If we have not let ourselves be misled by the methodological traps mentioned before, and have observed a real placebo effect, what could the operating mechanisms be? What becomes clear is that placebo effects result from an interplay of different factors on different levels, in which mutual causality (interactions) and feedback may be supposed to operate. At least the following levels are involved.

Table 1: Overview of determining factors in the placebo effect

Biological variables
• psychoneuroimmunological reactions on transfer of information • body-mind interactions • transfer of (weak emission, subtle) energies • learned conditional reflexes

Patient variables
• type of illness (including psychiatric disorders) • suggestibility • the personal reaction to the stimulus of the placebo • learning and socialisation • expectations about treatment • characteristics like age, sex, intelligence • patterns in and stage of inner development • anxiety • faith and hope • personality traits • mind-body relationship • somatization • victim/participatorship in life • defense mechanisms • motivation • meaning • guilt dynamics • unconscious processes • self-concept • level of experienced stress • dreams, inner images, fantasies • conditioning of the intake of certain pills (intake rituals) • positive expectation in relationship to the substance • attitude vis-a-vis medical authorities • loneliness

Situational variables
• treatment procedures • size, color and shape of tablets or capsules • social and physical context of treatment (e.g., clinic, GP practice or laboratory) • general life conditions of the patient • influence of other patients (exp. influence of treated on untreated patients).

Patient-Physician variables
• attitude of the physician towards his patient (interest, warmth, friendliness, neutrality, lack of interest, rejection, hostility, etc.) • empathic abilities of the therapist • transfer of attention, sympathy, status, etc. • redefinition of social roles • competence and ability of suggestive influencing by the therapist • authority of therapist, social prestige • (general) therapeutical competence • physician's expectation of improvement, and more general his attitude towards treatment (faith, belief, enthusiasm, conviction, commitment, optimism, positive and negative expectations, scepticism, disbelief, pessimism, etc.) • dominance – submission • conviction about the effectiveness of treatment • elicitation of catharsis • the theoretical frame of reference of the physician and his belief in it • the factual interaction between physician and patient • the physician's attitude towards his own competence: anxiety, feeling of guilt and inadequacy • communication of reassurance about fundamental fears and uniqueness "I'm allowed to be who I am".

Social relationships in which the patient lives
• quality of the partner relationship and family life • crises in relationships • loss of partner, or family members or friends• reactions of others on the treatment; acceptance or rejection of the sick role • quality of social and work relationships • quality of friendships • environmental changes

Although the list given here is extensive, it can hardly be complete. So many factors are of influence. It is impossible to discuss all these factors here. We select some major factors, as well as factors which lead us to new lines of research that could bring us additional explanations for the placebo effect in the future.

Influence of history
A placebo is always given in the context of the personal history of the patient. Former (positive or negative) experiences with medicaments, socialisation and learning processes, cultural views on medicine, etc., will all be influential.

Symbolic transformations of reality
To give a placebo can elicit many transformations of reality. It can first mobilize a positive "belief system." The belief in the remedy and in the healer (or in something else) seems to mobilize powerful innate self-healing mechanisms within a person (Ornstein & Sobel 1987: 77). The belief system is also dependent upon the reaction and belief system of the therapist. It is a mutually reinforcing system: *"The patient can depend on the therapist's integrity and competence, and be supported by the belief that he will be helped. The more intense the belief of the therapist in his treatment, the more impressed will be the patient and the greater his belief"* (Shapiro 1971: 457). Secondly, offering a placebo changes definitions of the situation by suggestions and by introducing self-fulfilling prophecies (see, e.g., the Hawthorn effect). Thirdly, receiving a placebo treatment can induce new meaning in life. Research in the field of psychotherapy reveals how important this factor is. Many diseases are influenced by it, and especially the experience of pain and suffering (Kaplun 1992). Last, but not least, applying a placebo treatment enables the therapist to give a new position to the patient within the current culture. The effect of the cultural context that produces profound symbolic meanings, often remains unnoticed. We are not aware of it, just as fishes are not aware of the water they swim in. Anthropologists have proven that usually a treatment consists of rituals in which the patient is placed within the cultural order.[5]

Transformations of the emotional household
Our culture is quite rationalistic and consequently pays too little attention to the emotional inner world of patients. The structure of the emotional inner world, I will call, according to Elias (1983), "the emotional household." Placebos, just

---

[5] For an analysis of this highly hidden symbolic "universe," see, for example, Psychiatrist Jerome Frank as quoted by Ornstein & Sobel 1987: 75-76.

like every meaningful action toward a person, can influence the inner world tremendously and quite instantly. Meditation exercises can show how immediately emotions change. A placebo can be accompanied by messages of hope able to turn depressive into more optimistic feelings, which by the mutual influence of the body-mind relationship, can turn down a process of illness. I would also like to mention what I call *the transfer of "energetic qualities"* (like empathy, values, sympathy, love, etc.). All kinds of emotion are transferred in the interaction between physician and patient, which transform the inner emotional household of a person. The patient feels as if s/he gets more "energy," or the reverse in case of a nocebo: If s/he cannot mobilize energy anymore, s/he is tired, depressive, etc.

Energetic transformations
Scientists hold a strange idea that all energetic forces in the world would already be known. I am convinced that this is a great illusion. It blocks the development of more innovative research. Current research shows the possibility of transfer of so far unknown types of energies or even the transfer of information without any material carrier. I can refer here to Sheldrake's morphogenetic fields (Sheldrake 1981), the weak energies emissions of Popp (Goodwin 1992), the work of Madeleine Bastide covering the transfer of information to the immune system (see elsewhere in this book), the advances in electroacupuncture, etc.[6] There is much serious work about energetic transformations, and one must consider the possibility that the results of this kind of research would offer additional explanations for some observed placebo effects.

Biographical development
There is much evidence that certain inner developments have a great impact on health and illnesses. Unfortunately, for many reasons the research in this field is still not very advanced. Especially we lack a solid biographical methodology to observe and investigate these themes (Lafaille & Lebeer 1991, Lafaille, Lebeer & Mielants 1995, Lafaille & Wildeboer 1995). Inner development is to a certain extent related to inner images which show themselves in dreams, fantasies, imagery, meditations. Its precise relationship to developmental processes is still largely unclear, but investigators with experience in this field do not doubt the presence of such a relationship. The best way to explain an inner process is to

---

6 Also the possibility of what is genuinely called "paranormal energies" must be considered, although I am more than sceptical about much of the literature in this field.

show it with an example. I take the example of one of my friends described by Weil in his scientific bestseller *Spontaneous Healing*. It is the example of a patient with a malignant tumour, who recovered completely after a deep spiritual crisis (the case of Mr. Terayama in Weil 1992: 100-103).The example shows an inner development that started as a person who is "victim" of his illness. The illness is experienced as something that comes from the outside, on which he cannot exert any control. Later, the illness was the carrier of a liberation of authority process and a pathway to deep spiritual experiences.

I do not want yet to go into a discussion about the aetiology of cancer. There is still a lot unknown. However, I want to use my friend's biography as a hypothetical example. If these kinds of processes do not play a part in cancer, in many other illnesses they do. So a main question for future research will be, how these kinds of processes relate to the placebo effect.

Social relationships
Since the end of the sixties, systems theory – especially the branch of it that gave birth to family therapy – showed the complexity of social relationships and how illnesses can be a reflection of and be influenced by these relationships (Mielants and Rijnders 1992). Because of the complexity of these kinds of relationships, there is a lack of good research in this field. In most medical research social relationships are put aside. Highly improperly. The role that social relationships play in placebo reactions has to be given much more attention than the literature shows now.

With the help of structural equation models, we can empirically investigate the influence of all the different factors mentioned above and their interrelationships. The following scheme is an illustration of such an approach (see figure 3). In principle, such a hypothetical scheme can be tested with Lisrel models, or (partly) with loglinear models.

To figure 3 the remark has to be added that some arrows can be replaced by double arrows showing mutual causal influence. Also, the possibility of influence of a factor on itself is put aside in the figure because this would make the figure too complex. Besides, there are nearly statistical models that allow to investigate empirically self-referential causalities. Nevertheless, there are good arguments to support the idea that such causalities are operating in placebo effects.

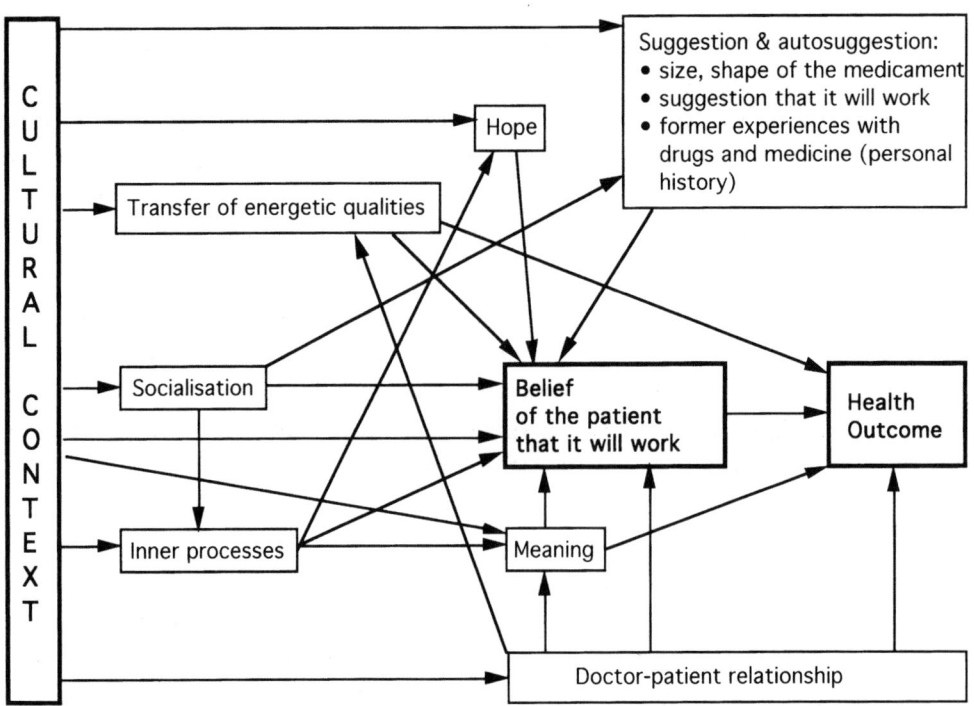

Figure 3: Path diagram of the determinants of a placebo effect

Historical Research as an Additional Instrument to Understand the Placebo Effect

Besides what I discussed so far, there are still other methods to get insight into how a placebo operates. Cross-cultural, anthropological and historical research can be mentioned here. I present one example of historical research to illustrate how symbolic transformations of reality function. Historical research has the advantage of contentual distance; one is not focused (as is a normal reaction in our culture) on the instrumental side of the treatment. One can investigate treatment methods that, according to the current medical knowledge, have no scientific basis. The total effect then has to be ascribed to placebo effects. If there are indications that patients are cured in relationship to these medical drugs or methods, one can look for explanations for these positive changes. This research topic cannot be investigated by the current mainstream of quantitative methods.

We made a thorough analysis of the Regimen of Salerno (Lafaille & Hiemstra 1990), a 12th or 13th century text of advice on a healthy life style that disseminated the medical knowledge of the School of Salerno to a popular audience. The theoretical background of the Regimen is humoural pathology. In historical respect, it is the most important Regimen in Western civilization. Our analysis was highly based upon insights about placebo phenomena.

What strikes us perhaps most from the modern scientific point of view, is the lack of accuracy and precision of the health model of the Regimen. This leads us to a main characteristic of the Regimen: it is multi-interpretable. Although the categories employed are of a very concrete nature, the relationships between them are in practice difficult to interpret and subject to manifold interpretations. Because of this there is room for placebo-medicine, i.e., medicine that uses the power to transform the definitions of reality as its main instrument. What kinds of symbolic transformations of reality are suggested by the Regimen? Which synchronous transformations of the emotional-experiential world are induced? Every ideology finds its concrete form in a rhetorical system, which I will call rhetoric. To understand the working of the symbolic transformations that the Regimen generates, some further explanation of this rhetoric is necessary. Every rhetoric system intends to give an explanation of reality (or a part of it) and has the tendency to encompass the whole reality. Some rhetorics even succeed inclusion of their own counterpart system or the denial of its legacy. The rhetoric of the Regimen is mainly a particular concretisation of the humoural pathological ideology. It is a very inclusive system that intends to encompass that part of reality related to health and illness (and perhaps more than that). The first symbolic transformation of reality that originates from this is that illness and discomfort are stripped of their daily personal significance, and interpreted as a distortion of the humoral household. Subsequently the discussion about health and illness is elevated to this level (instead of the level of body sensations). In other words the rhetoric of the Regimen leads the patient away from his own definitions of his own body experience and replaces this by an ideological construct. Once the rhetoric has been accepted, important emotional transformations appear: tranquillity, security and consolation. By an interpretation of health and illness from a socially constructed, but therefore generally accepted framework, health and illness are transformed from an individual to a social fact. Individual experiences become, through the mediation of the rhetoric system, communicable to others. This mediation also supplies new definitions of the situation (for the persons themselves and their social environment simultaneously), and possibly – in severe or life threatening disorders – a new social role. The all encompassing character of the rhetoric not only offers the questioning mind tranquillity and intellectual satisfaction, but the social processes started by it also offer tranquillity and consolation. The rhetoric also brings a great amount of security, which is even amplified by the decisive style of writing: Things are clear, and if you do the right things your health will be ensured. For all kinds of situations there are explanations and solutions. Highly developed rhetorics are characterized by the fact that they offer an explanation for everything. Humoural pathology represents such a kind of highly developed rhetoric: Thus, earache was explained by the excessive pressure of phlegm from the brain on the ears; and sperm was also supposed to be composed of phlegm, which is transported from the spinal marrow to the penis; and the increase of phlegm in the blood during pregnancy was explained by the assumption that it was the function of menstruation to provide for the removal of phlegm, and that during pregnancy menstruation ceased to come (Van Dijk 1981: 36-37). A second series of transformations refers to what one, analogous to the humoural household, might call the emotional household. How does the Regimen influence the emotions? To answer this question, I will first turn back to the text itself. In the text there are regular references to emotions (sadness, pain, passion, etc.), but mostly concerning the corporal side of processes that encompass an emotional component: The production of semen, swelling, a soft abdomen, trembling of the hands. Somatization was already in fashion then.

To establish the equilibrium of the emotional household, two lines of thought are presented; each of them is valid separately, but also in combination (which heightens their multi-interpretability).

The first line puts forward that an equilibrium in the emotional household can be reached by following the right diet. Examples among others are:

• the fig generates lice and lust • vinegar has more of a drying effect: it cools, makes a man thin, induces melancholy, decreases the number of sperm, harms those of dry humour, and dries up the nerves of the fats • very salty foods hurt the eyes and decrease sperm • certain flavors temper feelings • sage calms the nerves and takes away hand tremors • rue gives keen eyesight, it influences sexual desire, makes chaste, intelligent and cunning • nettle gives sleep • chervil cuts off pain, it often stops vomiting and loose bowels • saffron makes cheery

The only exception possibly to this rule is (because the role of sharp eyes is not clear) that washing sharpens the eyes. Even fluctuations of mood are caused by the diet and by the humoural household that is related to that diet: "In autumn beware that fruits do not become cause for mourning. Add the flower of the rose and it will strongly diminish your love."

It is typical of the Regimen that it establishes a one-sided relationship between diet and the inner experiential world of people. No interdependent relationship is supposed to exist between emotions/consciousness and nutrition. The outside world is decisive for the inner world. This leads us to the possibility to intervene from the outside into the inner world (the world of human experience), and especially by changing the nutritional habits through diet. In principle this also leads to the opportunity of an external manipulation of feelings (as in our century especially psychiatry and more precisely bio-psychiatry tries to do).

The second line of thought refers to the four humoural temperaments that would determine the experiences of the individual. Because the diet influences the mixture of humours, both lines of thought can easily be combined; in the text they are permanently confused.

Besides diet, venesection is the most favourite instrument for the regulation of emotions. From such a point of view a similar "medieval" practice gets completely different significance than it represents on face-value. That venesection influences emotions is clearly shown in the text of the Regimen. Certain effects are listed: that sadness changes into cheerfulness, that anger is turned into tranquillity, and that sexual impulses decline. Even the exact time at which venesection should be applied, is clearly connected with emotions, namely when you become irritable. Would not the intention be here that "when the barrel of emotions is full" one can by venesection "blow off steam?" It will be evident that venesection interferes in the experiential world of the person and that symbolic and emotional transformations will appear. The application of venesection implies: 1) On the symbolic level that the condition of the body and its definitions are stripped of their daily meaning and translated into the terminology of humoural pathology (blood, corporal humours); 2) on the emotional level, that substitution of emotion arises. The initial feelings of discomfort caused by (or in psychosomatic disorders: source of) the illness are replaced by the pain of the venesection itself and other emotions induced by the ritual of venesection. With an age-long practice of venesection as a background, the hypothesis is legitimate that this practice was so longstanding because venesection was a very effective instrument for the substitution of emotions.

Finally, it has to be underlined that in the Regimen venesection is much more than the introduction of an incision, but that this corporal intervention is incorporated in a ritual which takes some days. The person has to prepare himself in a certain manner, also emotionally (carrying out all instructions with care and attention) and after the introduction of the incision, he has to stay awake for six hours, he has to go without food for some time, no milk, no alcoholic drinks are allowed (they could arouse other feelings and emotions, and alcohol too is an already age-old instrument for the substitution of emotions!), he has to take care not to get cold, and he has to take a good rest.

My historical research has led to a redefinition of magical practices in a structuralistic manner, which might be a fruitful theoretical line for further historical research into the placebo effect. Magic can then be defined as *"every behavior that generates a symbolic transformation of reality which causes synchronic transformations of the emotional-experiential world of the individual and of the context in which the individual participates which forms the object of these 'magical' actions"* (Lafaille & Hiemstra 1990: 66). Such a definition opens magic for an interesting scientific investigation that retains an empirical nature.

Conclusions

Healing is a very special and wonderful phenomenon. Placebo research adds vital dimensions to more classical clinical research. Placebo as a scientific concept is accepted, but one has also to be cautious not to expand it to other domains than the pharmacological. Placebo research reveals a quite endless series of influencing factors. Moreover, applying a placebo itself causes placebo effects too, and research into the placebo effect its turn can create placebo effects. It is a quite complicated matter. For the human sciences, it is better not to introduce placebo as a *core* concept. I would suggest handling these matters in broader theories about healing. This offers a more appropriate perspective in which placebo research can have an adequate place.

As a scientist I would plead to promote placebo research. Why should not every medical faculty put placebo research on his research program? Is it not important enough? It counts on average for ± 30% of all health improvements (Martens 1984: 41). Moreover, with only a small investment to every testing of new medicaments, some topics from the field of placebo research can be added. Why do not medical faculties invest in this? It is low budget research. I think general practice has to take up this challenge, because they hold a position between hard medical interventions and guidance of patients and their families. They should become experts in using positive "placebo effects"! I would also hold a playdoyer that the human sciences would become more active in this field. On the political level I have a suggestion: Why not use the results of placebo research as a criterion to decide where to cut the costs of health care or how to reform therapeutical practices? If certain illnesses react highly on a placebo, other kinds of treatment have to be promoted to more than just prescribing "pills".

Acknowledgments

I am indebted to the following colleagues who inspired me or commented on a first draft of the text: Prof. Dr. Madeleine Bastide (France), Stud. Med. Toke Barfod (Denmark), Prof. Dr. Brian Goodwin (Open University UK), Drs. Hennie Hiemstra (Holland), Dr. Paul J. Lewi (Janssen Pharmaceutica, Belgium),

Dr. Guido Magnus (Belgium), Dr. Eveline Van Puyvelde (IIAHS, Belgium), and to all participants of the INRAT conference 1995 for their stimulating comments.

References

Bowman, W. C. and Rand, M. J.
    1980   *Textbook of Pharmacology*, Blackwell Scientific Publications: Oxford.

Brodeur, D.W.
    1965   "A short history of placebos", in: *J. Amer. Pharm. Assoc.*, 5: 642-662.

Buncher, C.
    1972   "Principles of Experimental Design for Clinical Drug Studies", in: D. E. Francke and H. A. K. Whitney (eds.): *Perspectives in Clinical Pharmacy*, pp. 504-525, Elsevier: New York.

Casti, J. L.
    1994   *Complexification. Explaining a Paradoxical World through the Science of Surprise*, Harper and Collins: New York.

Cousins, N.
    1977   "The mysterious placebo: How mind helps medicine work", in: *Saterday Rev.*, Oct.: 9-16.

Dessens, J. and Jansen, W.
    1982   "Terugval naar het gemiddelde; een methodologische notitie", in: *Sociologische Gids*, (56): 410-419.

Dijk, P. Van
    1979   *Geneeswijzen in Nederland* (Complementary Medicine in Holland), Ankh-Hermes: Deventer.
    1981   *Volksgeneeskunst in Nederland en Vlaanderen* (Folkmedicine in Holland and Flanders), Ankh-Hermes: Deventer.

Elias, N.
    1983   *Power and Civility. The Civilizing Process*, Pantheon Books: UK.

Evans, F.
    1967   "Suggestibility in the normal walking state", in: *Psychological Bulletin*, 67(2): 114-129.
    1974   "The placebo response in pain reduction", in: J. J. Bonica (ed.): *Pain. Advances in Neurology*, Raven Press: New York.

Fisher
    1970   "Nonspecific Factors in Response to Drugs", in: DiMascio and Shader (eds.): *Clinical Handbook of Psychopharmacology*, Williams & Wilkins: Baltimore.

Fulder, S.
    1987   *The Handbook of Complementary Medicine*, Coronet: London.

Geert, P. Van
    1991   "A Dynamic Systems Model of Cognitive and Language Growth", in: *Psychological Review*, 89(1): 3-53.

Goodman Gilman, A., Rall, T. W., Nies, A. S. and Taylor, P.
1992 *Goodman Gilman's the Pharmacological Basis of Therapeutics*, McGraw Hill: New York.

Goodwin, B.
1992 "Frontiers of Biology in Relation to Health", in: R. Lafaille and S. Fulder (eds.): *Towards a New Science of Health*, pp. 51-58, Routledge: London.

Jospe, M.
1978 *The Placebo Effect in Healing*, Lexington: Toronto.

Kaplun, A.
1992 *Health Promotion and Chronic Illness. Discovering a New Quality of Health*, Copenhagen: WHO Regional Publications, European Series, No. 44.

Kissel, P. and Burrucand, D.
1964 *Placebos et Effet Placebo en Medicine*, Masson: Paris.

Lafaille, R.
1989 "Empowerment of People: Unilateral Armament, Unilateral Disarmament or Bilateral Disarmament?", in: J. W. Salmon and E. Gopel (eds.): *Proceedings of the International Symposium "Community Participation and Empowerment Strategies in Health Promotion"*, Center for Interdisciplinary Research (ZIF), University of Bielefeld, June 5-9: Bielefeld.
1984 "Self-Help as Self-Care", in: S. Hatch and I. Kickbusch (eds.): *Self-Help and Health*, pp. 169-176, W. H. O.: Copenhagen.
1994 "Auf dem Weg zu einer Gründung der Gesundheitswissenschaften: Möglichkeiten, Herausforderungen, Fallstricke", in: E. Göpel and U. Schneider-Wohlfart (eds.): *Provokationen zur Gesundheit. Beiträge zu einem reflexiven Verständnis von Gesundheit und Krankheit*, pp. 229-266, Mabuse: Frankfurt/M.
1995 *Investigating Biographies: the Formulation of a Meta-Model*, International Institute for Advanced Health Studies: Antwerp.

Lafaille, R. and Fulder, S. (eds.)
1992 *Towards a New Science of Health*, Routledge: London.

Lafaille, R. and Hiemstra, H.
1990 "The Regimen of Salerno, a contemporary analysis", in: *Health Promotion International*, 1(5): 57-74.

Lafaille, R. and Lebeer, J.
1991 "The Relevance of Life Histories for Understanding Health and Healing", in: *Advances*, 4(7): 16-31.

Lafaille, R., Lebeer, J. and Mielants, P.
1995 *The Study of Life Histories for Understanding Health and Healing. The Observation of the Biographical process. Part A: Fundamental Issues*, International Institute for Advanced Health Studies: Antwerp.

Lafaille, R. and Wildeboer, H.
1995 *Validity and Reliability during the Process of Observation and Data Collection*, International Institute for Advanced Health Studies: Antwerp.
1996 *Biographical Methodology and Research*, Bibliography of the Health Sciences, Vol. 9, International Institute for Advanced Health Studies: Antwerp.

Lasagna, L., Mosteller, F. , Felsinger, J. and Beecher, H.
1954 "A study of the placebo response", in: *American Journal of Medicine*, (16): 770-779.

Mabeck, C. E.
1994 "Behandling", in: *Lægen og Patienten – Patient-Centreret Medicin i Teori og Praksis*, pp. 313-332, Munksgaard: Copenhagen.

Martens, F.
1984 "Effet Placebo et Transfer", in: *Psychoanalyse* (Belgian School for Psychoanalysis), 1(1): 38-62.

McDonald, C. J. and Mazzuca, S. A.
1983 "How much of the Placebo effect is really statistical regression?", in: *Stat. Med.*, 2: 417-427.

Mielants, P. and Rijnders, P.
1992 "Health at Social Crossroads", in: R. Lafaille and S. Fulder (eds.): *Towards a New Science of Health*, pp. 84-104, Routledge: London.

Ornstein, R. and Sobel, D.
1987 *The Healing Brain. Breakthrough Discoveries about how the Brain keeps us Healthy*, Simon and Schuster: New York.

Pfag, C. and Zelvelder, W.
1975 "Therapeutische waardebepaling van enkele analgetica en placebo", in: *Tijdschrift voor Geneesmiddelenonderzoek – Journal of Drug Research*, (Nov.-Dec.): 11-16.

No author
1975 "Placebo's", in: *Tijdschrift voor Geneesmiddelenonderzoek – Journal of Drug Research*, (Nov.-Dec.) 6-10.

Sanford, R. L.
1994 "The Wonders of Placebo", in: C. R. Buncher and J.-Y. Tsay (eds.): *Statistics in the Pharmaceutical Industry*, pp. 247-266, Marcel Dekker: New York, Basel and Hong Kong.

Schwartz, E. (ed.)
1985 *Placebo: Theory, Research and Mechanisms*, The Guilford Press: New York.

Shapiro, A. K.
1964 "A historic and heuristic definition of the placebo", in: *Psychiatry*, (27)1: 52-58.
1960 "A contribution to the history of the placebo effect", in: *Behav. Sci.*, (5).
1963 "Psychological use of medication", in: M. Lief (ed.): *Psychological Basis of Medical Practice*, Harper and Row: New York.
1971 "Placebo Effects in Medicine, Psychotherapy and Psychoanalysis", in: A. Bergin and S. Garfield (eds.): *Handbook of Psychotherapy and Behavioral Change*, Wiley: New York.

Sheldrake, R.
1981 *The New Science of Life*, Blond and Briggs: London.

Vinar, O.
1968 "A Discussion of the Appropriateness of Placebo Use in Psychotic Subjects", in: K. Rickels (ed.): *Nonspecific Factors in Drug Therapy*, Charles C. Thomas: Springfield.

Weil, A.
1995   *Spontaneous Healing. How to Discover and Enhance Your Body's Natural Ability to Maintain and Heal Itself*, Alfred A. Knopf: New York.

White, L. (et al)
1985   *Placebo, Theory, Research and Measurement*, The Guilford Press: New York.

Part IV

Researching and Networking

Research and Communication: The Work of the Research Council for Complementary Medicine

by Rebecca Rees

The Research Council for Complementary Medicine promotes and evaluates rigorous research in complementary medicine so as to encourage safe, effective practice and improved patient care.

Founded in the UK in 1983, the RCCM is an independent, charitable body. Our charity deeds demand that the organisation promotes rigorous research into all aspects of the various complementary therapies. We use various methods to promote research, methods that need monitoring and adapting as the field of complementary medicine research develops.

The Context: Complementary Medicine in the UK

In the British Isles, non-medically qualified practitioners of unconventional medicine are free to practice under common law. British osteopaths and chiropractors are now subject to statutory regulation and both will soon have a single register of practitioners. This Autumn, five British acupuncture societies will jointly form a single regulatory body, with statutory regulation as one of its first objectives.

Complementary medicine use is considerable. An unpublished 1993 survey (Thomas et al 1993), estimated that 8.5% of those interviewed (n=718) had visited a therapist of one of the big six therapies (acupuncture, osteopathy, chiropractic, homoeopathy, herbal medicine, hypnotherapy) in the previous 12 months. Estimated lifetime use was almost 20%. Other therapies will add to this total. Certain groups (e.g., those with chronic conditions) are likely to use complementary medicine more frequently than this average suggests.

A look at the history of the RCCM from 1983 to 1995 illustrates how the organisation has changed in response to a changing research climate.

Stage One: Fund-Raiser and Convenor

The RCCM initially worked mainly as a broker, raising funds and then distributing them to research projects. Over one million pounds have been distributed since 1983 for investigations varying from the use of Alexander technique for improving music performance, through a study of acupuncture for hypertension, to a pilot-scale study into the level of use of complementary therapies in the UK.

The organisation worked to build bridges between groups, holding conferences and seminars to bring researchers together to debate research issues. This work highlights the importance of the RCCM's role as a neutral body: neither for or against complementary medicine; not allied with any one particular therapy. The peer-reviewed journal, Complementary Medicine Research, was produced in-house. In 1993 the title was purchased by publishers Churchill Livingstone and renamed Complementary Therapies in Medicine. The journal remains the major peer-reviewed journal in its field.

The RCCM provides on-call advice to researchers about methodology and research design. The complementary medicine "methodology debate" has been a controversial one over the past 13 years, with much confusion over the appropriate use of various methodological safeguards (blinding and randomisation being two examples). The RCCM has worked to lessen this confusion through conferences and published work. We encourage researchers to focus on the question they hope to address. Using the RCCM's in-house bibliographic database, we can then provide practical examples of the research techniques that fit each question.

Stage Two: Consolidation

Over the past two years, the RCCM has moved away from funding primary research. In 1993, the British Medical Association published a report calling, amongst other things, for research in complementary medicine (BMA 1993). National and regional funding bodies now have a greater interest in supporting high quality research proposals, although still on a relatively modest scale. The RCCM has therefore become a service-based organisation that assists researchers and those interested in the results of research throughout the research process.

We now promote research by encouraging a research ethos within complementary medicine, assisting communication between researchers and making the results of previous research available. Four main projects have helped these aims.

Research education working party

It is generally recognised that students of the complementary therapies need to be familiar with the research base of their therapy. More importantly, it is generally agreed that it is important for practitioners of all kinds to have a questioning approach to their own practice: the idea of reflective practice.

The RCCM's research education working party has brought together representatives from 15 of the main training colleges in the UK. Some of these, notably some of the osteopathic and chiropractic colleges, have well established research centres and have research firmly on the student curriculum. Others do not teach research skills at all or merely horrify their students with short, sharp statistics courses: possibly killing the idea that research can be interesting for good.

The working party was set up as a forum for the exchange of skills, ideas and experience; again the RCCM's role was as a convenor. It was just as well that we did not set any agendas as we had imagined that the group might spend most of its time discussing what needed to go on the curriculum. Instead, the group spent a large amount of time discussing the interconnectedness of research and institutional development. The more developed schools had tales to tell of failed attempts that merely added research methods to student courses without investigating the relevance of research to the curriculum in general and the school as a whole.

Instead, they had learned that the importance of research and reflective practice needs to be understood by the entire faculty of a college and that resources need to be put behind this ideal. For instance, staff need to be supported to undertake postgraduate, research-based degrees; the school needs to support a full-time staff member to work solely on research teaching and development; money needs to be found for library facilities to support increased student interest.

The working party also acted as a forum for collaboration between those interested in the UK library resources for complementary medicine, most of which are situated for the training schools. A resource pack on literature searching within complementary medicine was produced. This is soon to be updated so as to add details of international bibliographic databases to the library and UK-based databases it already contains.

Several of the colleges involved with the working party have since invited RCCM staff members to give lectures introducing students to research. This has proved invaluable experience for us. We have been able to discuss with students why they think research is important, what research is, and what constitutes reliable information, along with more specific questions of research design and appraisal.

Some of these students will be the researchers of tomorrow. Some of them will carry out experimental research. However, if they go on to practice they will also need to become familiar with techniques that they can use to evaluate their own practice. This is another whole area of research that the RCCM is now working to promote.

"First Rung" awards for first-time researchers
These small grants of up to £2,500 per project are to encourage pilot-scale, simple research into complementary therapies by first-time UK-based researchers. The project aims not to produce research, as such, but to encourage a research ethos within the field. To be eligible, researchers must have suitable academic or institutional support. One winner of the 1994 awards, a professional homoeopath, worked in collaboration with researchers at the University of Oxford. She has since received "second-rung" funding from a larger funding body on the strength of her pilot work investigating homoeopathy for the treatment of autistic children.

Research network
Researchers in complementary medicine can be isolated. Research can take a long time to come to fruition and be published. The RCCM's research network aims to help researchers overcome some of these problems. The RCCM consists of a database of 740 ongoing research projects and individuals' interests. Researchers can carry out searches over the telephone to see who has registered in a research area.

This service is currently used mainly by those whose therapy organisations are less developed. For instance, aromatherapists and reflexologists are often glad to hear of other research-inclined fellow practitioners. A growing number of what are sometimes termed "innovative projects" are also accessible through the network. These are clinics where complementary therapies are being provided alongside orthodox general practice, or within the national health system. The network can also provide information regarding the methods and measures that are being used to evaluate practice outcomes and processes.

Bulletin
The RCCM's quarterly bulletin currently reaches 600 researchers internationally and provides updates of RCCM projects. It also contains overviews based on research papers found in the RCCM's CISCOM database. In a recent survey of readers this "research digest" was voted the most useful part of the bulletin. Future developments may include more detailed and more frequent updates of published work. The RCCM is already able to provide information overviews

rapidly by electronic means: Future mailings are likely to be tailored to fit individual researcher interests.

The CISCOM bibliographic database
Bibliographic searches are the first step in evaluating a therapy and form the basis of any research proposal. References to complementary medicine research are scattered over a variety of bibliographic databases. Each database indexes papers from a different set of journals: Medline, produced by the US National Library of Medicine, excludes many complementary medicine specific journals. Embase, a database published by Elsevier, contains many articles published in European journals that are not indexed by Medline. The British Library's AMED database inputs references from many of the relevant journals not covered by these other two databases but has several characteristics that make it hard to use.

The RCCM's in-house bibliographic database (CISCOM) combines data from these three sources with data sourced by hand searching and citation tracking. It contains 35,000 references to papers published worldwide from the 1960s onwards. CISCOM searches can be carried out with respect to journal and publication type.

CISCOM has been created to act as a centralised source of published information, with the ability to find "higher quality" data (e.g., systematic literature reviews, controlled trials and other controlled studies). Using CISCOM, researchers can see what has been studied in their area of interest and can examine previous methodology and identify suitable outcome measures for further research.

The RCCM currently handles approximately 100 information requests each month. Costs are covered by a search charge that starts at around £15 sterling. Search results can be distributed in printed or electronic format. The database can be accessed by phoning, faxing or emailing the RCCM. Searches will usually need to be negotiated with a quick telephone call, kept brief so as to reduce costs for overseas users.

Table 1 illustrates the number of papers held on CISCOM. The numbers shown are the results of a general search that specifies a selection of therapies and publication types. Basic research is here used to mean controlled studies in non-clinical settings. These might include, for instance, laboratory tests of an essential oil for its antimicrobial properties or experiments to examine the response in healthy volunteers to electroacupuncture at a suspected placebo acupuncture point.

The publication types shown here are the ones that are of greatest interest to most researchers. In addition to the types shown, the database holds the details of clinical case studies, historical references and social research studies, for instance, surveys of usage and attitudes.

Stage 3. The Future: Pragmatism

The context of the RCCM's work has changed considerably over its 13 years. Three ongoing projects in particular illustrate the organisation's most recent responses to the need for research-based information and communication in complementary medicine.

Familiarisation of medical students and practising doctors
It has been said that doctors need to be acquainted with complementary medicine simply because its use is commonplace. Medical students need to have at least a basic grasp of the various complementary therapies. The British Medical Association has called for programmes of familiarisation.

One recent survey of doctors in the Thames region (Perkin et al 1994) showed that 93% had referred to a complementary practitioner, 20% were practising a complementary therapy and 80-95% of trainee GPs claim that they want basic training in a complementary therapy.

A recent RCCM colloquium brought practitioners and representatives of medical colleges together to discuss this issue. A medical member of staff has been appointed to develop familiarisation projects at both the undergraduate and postgraduate medical level.

Systematic evaluation of research
The RCCM is also participating in the Cochrane Collaboration, an international grouping of individuals committed to collecting and disseminating the results of randomised controlled trials (RCTs). The organisation is represented within a Cochrane complementary medicine field. This grouping is establishing a register and archive of complementary medicine RCTs that will inform systematic reviews of research in specific health care areas as they arise.

Evaluation and audit of complementary therapies in practice
This research attempts to investigate aspects of therapy provision, as it is practised. The structure, process and outcomes of care need to be rigorously evaluated if health care providers are to be confident that they are caring for their patients effectively. The RCCM is currently developing a service to assist practitioners and health authorities in this area.

We are always interested in hearing from researchers working in complementary medicine. What would you like the RCCM to do to promote research in the field? Further information about the work of the Research Council for Complementary Medicine can be obtained by writing to the following address. RCCM, 60 Great Ormond Street, London WC1N 3JF. Telephone: 0044 0171 833 8897. Fax: 0044 0171 278 8897. Email: rccm@gn.apc.org.

References

British Medical Association
1993 *Complementary Medicine: New Approaches to Good Practice*, Oxford University Press: Oxford.

Perkin, M. R., Pearcy, R. M. and Fraser, J. S.
1994 "A Comparison of the Attitudes shown by General Practitioners, Hospital Doctors and Medical Students towards Alternative Medicine", in: *Journal of the Royal Society of Medicine*, 87(9): 523-5.

Thomas, K., Fall, M., Nicholl, J. and Willams, B.
1993 *Methodological Study to Investigate the Feasibility of Conducting a Population-based Survey of the use of Complementary Health Care*, Unpublished report funded by the Research Council for Complementary Medicine: London.

Table 1: *The number of bibliographic references held on the RCCM's CISCOM database October 1995: the results of a general search specifying a selection of therapies and publication types*

THERAPY   **PUBLICATION TYPE**

	Clinical trials	Randomised clinical trials	Basic research papers	Total number of records held
Acupuncture	428	(194)	409	3966
Homoeopathy	213	(98)	394	5962
Herbal medicine	559	(225)	353	6643
Osteopathy	9	(5)	10	543
Chiropractic	56	(39)	30	2366
Manipulative Therapy (unspecified)	51	(37)	15	874
Hypnosis	62	(48)	132	1931
Meditation/ relaxation	397	(161)	82	1385
Massage	88	(35)	90	433
Essential oils	57	(25)	175	555
Yoga	31	(12)	36	182
Healing	30	(16)	9	302
Reflexology	4	(4)	0	55
Nutrition	565		172	2996
Naturopathy	39	(21)	5	447
Talk therapies	114	(9)	0	384
Psychological intervention	707	(219)	163	4710
Nothing in therapy field	357	(124)	156	5248

Integration of Complementary Medicine in Research at the University of Munich

by Dieter Melchart

Complementary and alternative medical practices are frequently used throughout the world and are becoming increasingly accepted in mainstream medicine (Eisenberg et al. 1993, IKK-Bundesverband 1994, Spigelblatt 1994).

However, the effectiveness of many complementary and alternative therapies is highly controversial. Many universities and medical insurance companies are still sceptical of scientific bases of this diverse and inconsistent medical field. There is an extensive need for research and databases.

This article describes the activities of the 'Münchener Modell', a project for 'Integration of Natural Healing Procedures into Research and Teaching' at the Ludwig-Maximilians-University in Munich (Melchart 1993a, 1994a, Melchart et al. 1995a).

What is Complementary Medicine?

Before doing this there is a need to answer the question what is *complementary medicine*? At present there is no clear definition of complementary medicine. Various expressions are used, such as 'alternative medicine', 'unconventional methods', 'holistic medicine', 'natural healing procedures' etc. In different countries different terms are used and the same terms have different meanings even within the same country. In spite of controversial discussions also in Germany, the concept of the project is based on the following definition: 'Natural Healing Procedures' (NHP) actively include and employ self-regulatory processes in treatment (autoregulation). The diagnostic and therapeutic procedures follow the principle of stimulus response (Melchart 1993b). In the framework of such a definition, NHPs comprise a broad spectrum of methods ranging from so-called classical natural treatments such as physiotherapy to homeopathy and acupuncture. All the methods can be distinguished by their 'Intervention Factors':

    naturistic
    physical
    bioinformative.

'Naturistic' means that all remedies should have a naturistic origin, i.e., water, air, light and soil. These are the so-called 'classical naturopathic methods' like hydrotherapy, herbal medicine and Kneipp therapy. Physiotherapy is based on 'physical' intervention-factors like radiation, warmth, cold, pressure, pulling and torsion and is regarded as plausible and belonging to the framework of natural science. A third group can be characterized with the word *'bioinformative'*, including methods like homeopathy, kinesiology etc., which are based on a kind of information process in which a cybernetic stimulus is transmitted to the organism.

Objectives, History and Structure of the "Münchener Modell"

'Münchener Modell' is the shortened name of a model project at Munich University for the Integration of Natural Healing Procedures into Research and Teaching. Since 1989 the project has been financed by special funds from the Bavarian Parliament and affiliated with the Institute of Anesthesiology – and later on – Institute of Pharmaceutical Biology. Additional temporary funding for defined activities has been provided by foundations (i.e., Erich Rothenfußer Stiftung), the Federal Ministery for Research and Technology, and Industry. Its fundamental objectives are to integrate Complementary Medicine, or as it is called in Germany, Natural Healing Procedures (NHP) into research and teaching of mainstream medicine, and to establish an academic institution, including a central department for research methodology and the clinical representation of the most relevant NHPs.

At present, there are several infrastructural and conceptual obstacles for efficient research of complementary medicine at German universities. The most important obstacle is the lack of expert practitioners and patients suitable for complementary therapies within university clinics. Therefore, the project does not aim to establish a conventional infrastructure of a chair, but a kind of network, linking research facilities within the university, and experts in complementary medicine outside the university (clinics, practitioners).

The history of the project 'Münchener Modell' goes back to the organization of ring lectures beginning in 1977 and a student initiative filing an application for the establishment of an Institute of Empirical Therapeutics in 1982. The student group had no success; nevertheless, it increased the range of lectures and organized various scientific events. Practitioners, academics and students from Munich University founded a study group that systematized and organized teaching activities and performed research. The model experiment was approved by the Medical Faculty in 1988.

Table 1: History of the project 'Münchener Modell'

1982	student initiative applies for an 'Institute for Empirical Therapeutics'
1988	university project at Munich University (LMU) funded by the Bavarian Parliament
1989-92	one-year courses of Natural Healing Procedures for medical students
1992	Natural Healing Procedures become an obligatory subject matter for all German medical schools – emphasis of project activities shifts towards research
1996	Research Unit within the Department of Internal Medicine at the Central Hospital of the Technical University (TU) in Munich

The project is chaired by a full-time leader (Dr. D. Melchart). The director of the Institute of Pharmaceutical Biology (Prof. Dr. H. Wagner) has the status of an honorary leader. At present, a secretary and 11 scientific staff members are employed: 6 physicians, 1 biostatistician, 1 biologist, 2 medical technical assistants and 1 economist.

The project organization is warranted by the work of a *'Coordination Office'*. Within this 'core-unit' a *central project group* plans, designs and coordinates the project activities. A *clinical study group* for the field of immunomodulation is based in one of the networked hospitals and an *immunological laboratory* is run at the Institute of Pharmaceutical Biology. From next year onwards the project will run a *research unit* at the Medical Department of Internal Medicine (Prof. Dr. Classen) at the Technical University of Munich.

An *interdisciplinary working group* of local practitioners, clinicians, and researchers gives methodological input and works as a kind of internal audit and supervision group. An *external advisory board* consisting of reputed clinicians and researchers is supervising the research activities. Finally, the *supporting committee* is building up a lobby to support our objectives and activities on a political level.

Since autumn 1992, the main emphasis of the project was placed on developing a network of complementary clinics with extensive experience in the field of complementary medicine. The following institutions are active within the network of clinics:

1. First German Clinic for Traditional Chinese Medicine, Kötzting (Erste Deutsche Klinik für Traditionelle Chinesische Medizin), 76 beds, 6 German and 8 Chinese physicians; main indication: chronic pain.
2. Clinic for Complementary Medicine in Höhenkirchen near Munich (Spezialklinik Höhenkirchen für Naturheilverfahren bei München), 70 beds, 5 resident and 4 consiliary physicians, main indication: allergic diseases; complemen-

tary therapies used: phytotherapy, homeopathy, dietetics, active hyperthermia, physical and psychological therapies, manual medicine, acupuncture.
3. Waldhaus Clinic for Internal Medicine in Stadtbergen near Augsburg (Waldhausklinik Deuringen), 42 beds; 5 physicians; complementary therapies used: homeopathy, phytotherapy, dietetics, physical therapy.
4. District Hospital in Simbach, first German Model Clinic for Integrated Medicine (Kreiskrankenhaus Simbach, Erste Deutsche Modellklinik für eine ganzheitsorientierte Grundversorgung), 176 beds with departments for Cardiology and General Internal Medicine (9 physicians); Rheumatology (3 physicians), Psychosomatic Medicine (4 physicians) and Complementary Medicine (7 physicians); complementary therapies used: physiotherapy, acupuncture, dietetics, homeopathy. The hospital provides basic health care services.

Short distances of a maximum of two hours' drive allow intensive interaction between the clinics. A total of 360 beds are available for research and teaching. The fulfillment of the legal and economic requirements for the participation of the individual clinics was made possible through support by the Working Committee of the Bavarian Medical Insurance Companies and by the Bavarian State Ministry for Labour and Social Order.

Table 2: Structure of the 'Münchener Modell'

Project structure
- Central Project Group (located in two university departments; 5 academic staff members, 1 secretary)
- Clinical Study Group Immunomodulation (located at the network clinic Höhenkirchen; 3 physicians)
- Immunological Laboratory (located at the Institute of Pharmaceutical Biology; 2 medical technical assistants)
- Research Unit Technical University (located at the Department of Internal Medicine, Central University Clinic; 1 physician)

Supervising/supporting structures
- Interdisciplinary Working Group
- External Advisory Board
- Supporting Commitee

Associated structures 1: Network of Clinics
- District Hospital Simbach (176 beds)

- TCM-Clinic Kötzting (76 beds)
- Special Clinic Höhenkirchen (70 beds)
- Waldhaus Clinic (35 beds)

Associated structure 2
- Quality Circle of General Practitioners

As a second step, the project is establishing a research circle of about 25 *general practitioners* (GP) in the Munich area using mainly complementary methods. The integration of this circle should link different levels of medical services. For the proof of a long-term benefit of a treatment regime for the patients, it is crucial to involve the GPs as a source of information (besides the patient himself).

Teaching Activities

From 1989 to 1992 the project ran three 1-year pregraduate courses in complementary medicine for medical students. Teaching objectives were basic knowledge of Natural Healing Procedures (NHPs) regarding diagnostics, determining indications and contraindications for specific techniques, ability to communicate between conventional medicine and complementary medicine and acquisition of basic practical skills in at least one specific method. (For more details see references Melchart 1990 and 1993a, Melchart et al 1994a). Since 1992 the fundamentals of NHPs have been an obligatory part of the subject matter for the examination in undergraduate medical education. That means that students in all German Medical Schools have to pass a NHP examination and the faculties henceforth have to offer this education. Despite this development, NHPs are still inadequately represented in academic medicine, teaching and research. In recent years two chairs have been established in Berlin (Prof. M. Bühring) and Ulm (Prof. T. Peters); also integration projects for complementary medicine have been established at the universities of Munich, Erlangen and Heidelberg.

Since 1993 the educational activities of the project have focused on the quality assurance of postgraduate education for the recognized additional title of Natural Healing Procedures. The German Medical Association prescribes at least 4 weeks of basic courses covering a specified list of topics and 3 months of internship or practical work under the supervision of a physician licensed for postgraduate education in this area. The 4-week courses are commonly organized as lectures with a large number of participants.

Pilot instruments for assessing the effectiveness of the course have been tested. Appropriate techniques have to be further developed to determine to what extent a predefined learning objective has been achieved by the candidate. The test should examine theoretical knowledge, problem-oriented competence, and performance skills in practice (Melchart et al 1995b).

Conceptual Aspects Relevant for Research on Complementary Medicine

Before describing the research activities of the project in detail, conceptual characteristics and features of complementary medicine which have influence on the research approach and on methodological issues have to be discussed.

The following statement summarizes some typical attributes and common characteristics of complementary medicine which should have influence on methodological issues:

Complementary medicine follows an *'autonomy-oriented respectively autoregulative medical concept'*, i.e., the natural ability and capacity of the individual for self-regulation, self-organization and self-responsibility represent the basis of medical thought and treatment. Most of these therapies are aimed at health-preserving and health-improving processes for the individual; this demonstrates the emphasis of complementary medicine on *influencing the entire lifestyle* of clients and patients.

Most of the complementary therapies are used to treat patients with chronic diseases suffering from functional, relapsing and nonspecific problems. Throughout the course of their chronic careers patients begin paying more attention to their "being ill" rather than to the illness itself. The patients demonstrate more changes in their state-of-mind than in their state-of-health. For the assessment of disorders of psychological well-being it is necessary to use appropriate (patient self-rating) questionnaires. Supposing you get a reliable and valid measure for such phenomena the question still remains open what extent of change is relevant and desirable for the treatment.

Many methodological problems arise when trying to prove the relevance of preventive outcomes. This implicates epidemiological comparisons with observations over long periods of time using specific instruments for measuring short- and long-term behavioral changes with respect to the lifestyle.

Many forms of non-drug-treatment require particular manual skills by a therapist, usually more than prescribing a drug. As an example, the quality and results of acupunctural therapy depends almost entirely upon the experience and skills of the acupuncturist. In comparison, this is not the case for prescribing for, e.g., an analgesic headache. Consequently, the *competence of the therapist* should be identified, documented and taken into consideration when evaluating the benefit of a particular treatment.

Another aspect concerning complementary medicine is that the mainly pathogenetically-oriented pattern of thinking in classical medicine is supplemented by a more *phenomenological-descriptive and individualized approach* when making a diagnosis. Generally, accepted and applicable guidelines for taking a case history, for determining therapeutic progress, and for defining the goals of a treatment do not exist for complementary medicine. Illness is often seen as a 'positive' reaction by the human organism in response to a certain situation in life and is interpreted as a message, a signal or sign to change something in life. Examples also include fever, the formation of an abscess or a psychological disorder. These aspects have to be taken into consideration in the documentation and interpretation of complementary medicine. Most of the strategies show a polymodal approach comparable with modern pain therapy. This makes sense, because human beings organize life on several levels (i.e., reflex level, vegetative and behaviorial level, consciousness level). To each level a certain form of treatment can be applied, i.e., physical therapy, osteopathy, homeopathy and psychotherapy. Therefore, it is only possible to study 'total effects' of a combined treatment, instead of specific effects of an isolated method.

Further characteristics of complementary medicine are the often missing immediate results, i.e., the delayed onset of the healing effects of drug or non-drug therapies. This corresponds to the *often serial, repetitive use of particular methods*. This is based on the fact that complementary methods tend to employ low doses and weak stimuli. The therapeutic effects can often be seen only after repeated use which leads to a 'training' or 'normalization' of self-regulating processes.

Another characteristic of experience-based methods is the fact that they have already been a traditional part of the medical system for several centuries. So, a scientific rationale for these methods often has to be created after their dissemination. Normally, theoretically founded explanations should precede the introduction of a new therapeutical method into practice. Opposite to newly developed drugs or health technologies complementary medical practices are not systematically evaluated by basic and clinical research *before* they become introduced into medical practices, but become scientifically investigated *only if* they are used in health care to such an extent that evaluation of risks and benefits is mandatory. Randomized controlled trials are necessary to investigate efficacy and effectiveness. But as it will be impossible for ethical, methodological and financial reasons to evaluate all complementary medicine by randomized controlled trials, other research tools have to be developed and tested. Clinical observations often provide accurate information concerning long-term natural history and results of treatment. Therefore, the project tried to establish an instrument called 'scientific quality management (sQM)' which tries to integrate both the classical way of controlled clinical trials and the way of structured observation (see below).

Research Activities

Scientific Quality Management in a network of clinics using Complementary Medical Practices (CMP)

A project 'scientific quality management' (sQM) (Melchart and Weidenhammer 1996) has been conceptualized, implemented and piloted in a network of four clinics using CMP with the following objectives: to evaluate structural characteristics (patients, clinic resources), processes (interventions) and outcomes (improvement of specific complaints, morbidity, quality of life); to develop guidelines; to optimize the ratio of patient-oriented utility, risks and costs.

A basic requirement for common quality assurance is the existence of an approved standard or guideline with which the result of intervention is compared. In complementary medicine there is a lack of such standards. In consequence, quality assurance is not possible in many fields of complementary medicine.

Scientific Quality Management (sQM) consists of the components "Quality Management" and "Attendant Scientific Research" (Melchart and Weidenhammer 1996). Within the sQM project a number of different study designs (including randomized trials) will be used, the main emphasis, however, will be on a prospective 'basic' documentation of all patients admitted to the clinics.

The basic documentation has been piloted in one of the networked hospitals, the Clinic for Traditional Chinese Medicine in Kötzting/Bavaria (manuscript submitted for publication). For all 1597 patients admitted and discharged between February 1992 and August 1993, diagnoses (western and Chinese), general prognostic factors (duration of disease, number of pretreatments) and interventions were documented. Physicians assessed changes at discharge. Patients were asked to assess the intensity of their main complaints (measured on a scale ranging from 1 = no complaints to 10 = intolerable complaints) at admission, at discharge, after 2, 6 and 12 months (postal follow up). Most patients suffered from different forms of chronic pain, the most common ICD diagnosis being migraine (n = 244). 64.5 % of all patients suffered more than 5 years from the main complaints. Mean intensity was 7.0 (n = 1551) at admission, 4.6 (1544) at discharge, 4.9. after 2 months (1338), 5.4 after 6 (1252) and 5.5 (1114) after 12 months. The pilot study showed that documentation of all patients is feasible, but especially outcome assessment has been too simplistic.

In the meantime a comprehensive case report method has been implemented. Outcome measurement includes intensity of main complaints, quality of life (instruments: POMS, MLDL, Alltagsleben) as well as indicators for morbidity and use of health care services. To ensure a valid and reliable documentation of potential side effects, a special report form has to be filled out and signed at discharge for every patient by the responsible physicians.

Several studies have been performed to investigate reliability and validity of our instruments. For the most frequent diagnoses (migraine, atopic dermatitis) in two clinics additional case report methods including clinical standard assessment methods are actually piloted.

At present the schedule shown in figure 1 is used for basic documentation in the networked clinics.

	Data source	Admission	Discharge	2 months after	6	12 admission
Basic biographic data of the patient; previous therapy, intensity of main complaint etc.	Pat	X				
Medical anamnesis, supposed therapeutical effectiveness	Phy	X				
Quality of Life Questionnaires (mood, satisfaction, everyday-life functional impairment)	Pat	X	X	X	X	X
Intensity of main complaint, satisfaction with therapy, concomitant therapies	Pat		X	X	X	X
Evaluation of therapeutical effectiveness concerning main complaints, final diagnosis	Phy		X			
Diagnostic/therapeutic services	Nur	X------->	X			
Pat=Patient Phy=Physician Nur=Nurse						

Figure 1: Schedule for the basic documentation in the network of clinics

To improve the comparability among the 4 clinics and different complementary practices, a standard set of guidelines for case taking is under development. Continuous feedback is warranted by quality circles in each of the network clinics.

As a second step, we are establishing a research circle of about 25 general practitioners in the Munich area using mainly complementary methods. The integration of these circles should enable us to interconnect different levels of medical services. For long-term observational studies, it is necessary to involve the assessment of general practitioners.

Several randomized clinical trials are in preparation to complete the sQM project. In the Clinic for TCM in Kötzting a trial comparing the effectiveness of acupuncture, sumatriptan and placebo for preventing migraine attacks is in the state of implementation. For this study a grant by the Federal Ministery of Education and Research could be approved.

Further randomized trials on the effect of lymph-drainage in migraine and acupuncture in gastroscopy are in the state of protocol development as well as a diagnostic trial on the usefulness of manual techniques for detecting patients with extrathoracal pain undergoing unnecessary coronary arteriography.

Evaluation of literature

The evaluation of the existing research evidence on complementary medicine is another research focus of the project. The project holds its own database of research publications and is involved in activities to integrate a 'Field Complementary Medicine' into the Cochrane Collaboration, a worldwide network with the objective to perform, continuously update and disseminate systematic reviews of RCTs in all relevant areas of health care (Godlee 1994). Systematic reviews – reviews based on a predefined research protocol describing literature search, selection, assessment and summarizing of results – have become the standard method for research synthesis in the last decade.

The project has undertaken systematic reviews on toxicological experiments and overviews of homoeopathy (Linde et al. 1994a and b) and herbal remedies (Melchart et al. 1994b). Actually, we are completing further reviews on the clinical trials of homoeopathy, acupuncture for asthma and St. John's word *(Hypericum)* for depression.

The experiences collected in the reviews have led to a number of methodological articles and recommendations for future research and its presentation (Linde et al. 1994c and d).

Research on immunomodulation

Immunomodulation by herbs and other preparations of natural origin has been a traditional research topic of the 'Münchener Modell' since its beginnings. The main objectives of these studies were to investigate the effects of extracts of echinacea (Melchart et al. 1995c), isolated polysaccharide fractions from echinacea (Melchart et al. 1993) and an extract from the thymus gland of calves (unpublished) on the phagocytosis of polymorphonuclear granulocytes and other immunofunctions. Studies on chronobiological influences on the immune systems of healthy volunteers were also undertaken (Melchart et al. 1992). A randomized double-blind clinical trial on the prevention of upper respiratory tract infections is just being analyzed, and an open study on immunomodulatory effects of an

Echinacea polysaccharide in cancer patients' echinacea is in progress.

In addition, a study on the effects of bacterial vaccines in patients with atopic dermatitis and immunological disorders is running.

Outlook

The final objective of the project is to make complementary medicine scientifically communicable and part of the scientific world. This is only possible if complementary medicine is open to criticism, able to admit errors, avoids ideological character and learns to play the rules of natural sciences (Sachverständigenrat 1992). The 'Münchener Modell' might be a pragmatic and efficient way to achieve an organized dialogue between these parties in order to obtain more benefit for the patient in future.

Mainstream medicine – on the other side – has to be more tolerant and should reflect more critically their own methodological approach to the field of complementary medicine.

References

Eisenberg, D. M., Kessler, R. C., Foster, C., Norlock, F. E., Calkins, D. R. and Delbanco, T. L.
    1993   "Unconventional medicine in the United States – prevalence, costs, and patterns of use", in: *New Engl J Med*, 328: 246-52.

Godlee, F.
    1994   "The Cochrane Collaboration", in: *Br Med J*, 309: 969-970.

IKK-Bundesverband
    1994   *Akzeptanz von Naturheilverfahren – Ergebnisse einer bundesweiten Repräsentativbefragung im Auftrag des IKK-Bundesverbandes*, IKK: Bergisch-Gladbach.

Linde, K., Jonas, W. B., Melchart, D., Worku, F., Wagner, H. and Eitel, F.
    1994a   "Critical review and meta-analysis of serial agitated dilutions in experimental toxicology", in: *Hum Exp Tox*, 13: 481-492.

Linde, K., Melchart, D., Brandmaier, R. and Eitel, F.
    1994b   "Critical evaluation of papers reviewing controlled clinical trials in homoeopathy", in: *Br Homoeopath J*, 8(3): 167-173.

Linde, K., Melchart, D., Jonas, W. B. and Hornung, J.
    1994c   "Ways to enhance the quality and acceptance of clinical and laboratory studies in homoeopathy", in: *Br Homoeopath J*, 83: 3-7.

Linde, K., Melchart, D. and Jonas, W. B.
1994d   "Durchführung und Interpretation systematischer Übersichtsarbeiten kontrollierter Studien in der Komplementärmedizin", in: *Forschende Komplementärmedizin*, 1: 8-16.

Melchart, D.
1990   "Integration von Naturheilverfahren in die Medizinerausbildung am Beispiel des Münchener Modells", in: *Therapeutikon*, 4: 502-505.
1993a   "Integration von Naturheilverfahren in Forschung und Lehre", in: *Therapeutikon*, 7: 99-107.
1993b   "Terminologie", in: D. Melchart and H. Wagner (eds.): *Naturheilverfahren – Grundlagen einer autoregulativen Medizin*, pp. 2-25, Schattauer: Stuttgart.
1994   Research in Complementary Medicine (Natural Healing Procedures) at the Munich Model in Germany, Abstracts of the First Methodology Conference of the NIH Office of Alternative Medicine, July 11-13.

Melchart, D., Martin, P., Hallek, M., Holzmann, M., Jurcic, K. and Wagner, H.
1992   "Circadian variation of the phagocytic activity of polymorphonuclear leukocytes and of various other parameter in 13 healthy male adults", in: *Chronobiol Internat*, 9: 35-45.

Melchart, D., Worku, F., Linde, K., Flesche, C., Eife, R. and Wagner, H.
1993   "Erste Phase-I-Untersuchung von Echinacea Polysaccharid (EPO VIIa/EPS) bei i.v. Applikation", in: *Erfahrungsheilkunde*, 42: 318-323.

Melchart, D., Worku, F., Linde, K. and Wagner, H.
1994a   "The university project Münchener Modell for the Integration of Naturopathy into Research and Teaching at the Ludwig-Maximilians University in Munich", in: *Comp Ther Med*, 2: 147-153.

Melchart, D., Linde, K., Worku, F., Bauer, R. and Wagner, H.
1994b   "Immunomodulation with Echinacea – a systematic review of controlled clinical trials", in: *Phytomedicine*, 1: 245-254.

Melchart, D., Linde, K., Weidenhammer, W., Worku, F. and Wagner, H.
1995a   "The integration of natural healing procedures into research and teaching at German universities", in: *Alternative Therapies*, 1: 30-33.

Melchart, D., Weidenhammer, W. and Perkuhn, K.
1995b   "Zur Situation der ärztlichen Weiterbildung in Naturheilverfahren: Beispiele europäischer Länder und eines Qualitässicherungsprojektes", in: *Forsch Komplementärmed*, 2: 203-210.

Melchart, D., Linde, K., Worku, F., Sarkady, L., Holzmann, M., Jurcic, K. and Wagner, H.
1995c   "Results of five randomized studies on the immunomodulatory activity of preparations of Echinacea", in: *J Alt Compl Med*, 1: 145-160.

Melchart, D., Weidenhammer, W.
1996   "Wissenschaftliches Qualitätsmanagement (wQM) und Naturheilverfahren – Definition, Aufgaben – und Problemstellung", in: J. Hornung (ed.): *Methodologie klinischer Studien in der Komplementärmedizin*, Schattauer: Stuttgart.

Sachverständigenrat der konzertierten Aktion im Gesundheitswesen
1990

Spigelblatt, D., Laine-Ammara, G., Pless, I. B. and Guyver, A.
1994   "The use of alternative medicine by children", in: *Pediatrics*, 94: 811-1814.

Communication, Publication and Information Opportunities on Computer Networks

– can scientific and therapeutic communities come closer together in cyberspace?

by Tobias Waltjen

Wednesday two weeks ago I went with a pile of paper to a Vienna medical publisher to have it proofread and afterwards published as a book. Proofreading will take 3 weeks, I was told, and then it may take at least another 3 weeks to do the printing. So, by the end of October, hopefully, we come out with the book, and of course, we hope to sell a lot of copies. Should you be one of our customers, however, you will have to wait another one to several weeks until the book is delivered to your place with the post.

Thursday one week ago I went to a friend who operates an Internet server in Vienna. I had with me a floppy disk with approximately 150 pages of text of our book, neatly reformatted to HTML, the language of the World Wide Web. After a short check that all the links worked, the files were copied to the World Wide Web server, a machine next door to the friend's office – and within a moment 150 pages were published worldwide.

"Published worldwide" means that everybody in the world with an Internet account has 24 hours, 365 days access to the pages, may look at them, save some of them to a local computer and send E-mail with further inquiries, corrections and so on to me from within the document being perused. At costs of a local telephone call – or cost free, in case a university or company account can be used.

Let me start with this real-world example for the current transition from traditional publishing to on-line publishing to discuss in some detail the question: Can scientific and therapeutic communities come closer together in cyberspace? I shall begin with the problems of

Communication in Scientific and Therapeutic Communities

Experience and knowledge are the sources of *what* we communicate and the fact that both are gained by individuals (as opposed to groups) is the reason *why* we wish to communicate.

Where does medical knowledge and experience come from? Doctors, therapists and nurses treat their patients, talk and listen to them, observe them and record the course of patients' diseases. By that, experience is gained. Experience is an ability to do something (medical treatment, therapy). Experience is also an ability to recognize the state of a patient from his or her appearance (diagnosis). Appearance has, in modern biomedicine, turned into clinical data obtained by means of physical and chemical, that is – scientific – methods which get their meaning within a framework of biomedical theory and empirical knowledge. But "appearance" in historical medicine and in complementary medicine means a total, integrated experience – and a personal experience, something that happens within one's mind.

Personal experience is not yet science. In fact it might not even be language. If an experienced person starts to talk about how she or he came to know or understand something, it will probably be a mixture of scientific concepts or concepts of one of the complementary medicine traditions and the person's private language. In scientific communities such a mixture is called laboratory slang and academic teachers spend a lot of time weeding out all the laboratory slang from their less experienced student's papers.

What I want to point out by this is: The transformation of one's own therapeutic experience into something that can be communicated is *work*. It needs training, it takes time, and in most cases the product can't be sold. Training in scientific work and publishing is not part of the curriculum for medical doctors (not to mention nurses and therapists) in Austria – unless a clinical career is chosen. Writing scientific papers for journals is out of reach for most members of medical professions. Members of medical professions tend to be busy treating patients. No time to sit down and chew a pencil staring at an empty piece of paper.

But members of medical professions do communicate: They give lectures and listen to lectures. Personal education is the preferred means for exchanging experiences – for several reasons:

1. Lectures are paid.
2. Spoken words don't need to be as precise, concise and systematic as written text (especially scientific papers).
3. Since therapeutic experience is something very personal – especially so in complementary medicine, as I mentioned earlier – a person teaching or giving a lecture tells you more than the words she or he is actually telling you. This extra-information is valuable and it is valued.

There are three other obstacles to communication in complementary medicine therapeutic and scientific communities:

1. Geographically scattered and therefore isolated communities. Everywhere on this planet (to put it a bit too simply) we find individuals, groups and institutions working with complementary medicine. But nowhere are the populations dense.
2. Language barriers and cultural barriers. Biomedicine has to a great extent internationalized use of English as *lingua franca*. Within complementary medicine we deal with a multitude of medical traditions, connected to different cultural traditions (Chinese, Indian, pre-scientific European) and different languages. Consequently communication services for complementary medicine face problems of semantics (nomenclature) and translation. On account of their nature those barriers cannot be broken down once and for all. Only repeated attempts to cross them will lower them.
3. Other barriers: scientific vs. alternative medicine, competing medical societies, and so on. Sometimes I wonder whether the main cause of poor communication is the unwillingness of the partners in the process to talk to each other. It is beyond the scope of a treatise on communication *means* to deal with this, but obviously the need for communication defines the market for information providers and communication services. So it is healthy to keep this point in mind.

Coming back to the cyberspace issue, we can draw the conclusion that if telematics (telecommunication plus computers) is to ease communication problems in complementary medicine, it has to meet the following expectations:

1. allow for (but no need for) the intellectual acrobatics of scientific publishing,
2. be time-saving,
3. be cost-saving,
4. be at least an indirect opportunity to earn money.

To Technical Obstacles there is a Technical Solution

How do the solutions look that are available for example on the Internet (which is today, but may not be forever, the most important and popular way of on-line communication and information)?

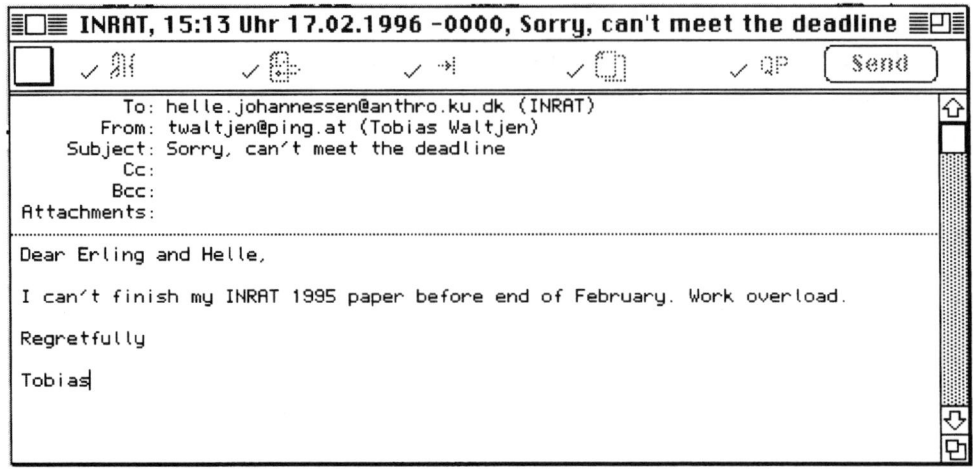

An Internet Mail Form (another real-world example)

Mail

An internet mail form contains a header with a title of message, name and E-mail addresses of the sender, the recipient(s), and the recipients of virtual carbon copies, whose names and addresses may be visible (Cc) or invisible (Bcc) to the recipients. The body may contain text you wish to quote from another letter (or from anywhere else), text that is a quote of a quote and so on, and new text. At the end of a message you can have a so-called signature automatically added on the bottom of a letter, containing name, affiliation and a motto (slogan) of the sender. (It is an equivalent to the printed letterhead on paper letters.) The opportunity to quote without rewriting has created a new style of letter writing: You quote the whole letter you want to answer and then just make annotations.

I mention these technical details, that you may be very familiar with, to make some points regarding the psychology of E-mail: E-mail forms are suitable to both formal and informal letters. They are an electronic equivalent to a post-it note (sticky note) with "Hi darling, I'm in the cinema tonight. Might come late. Sorry, Love" and to a formal letter with letterhead, text nicely placed on the page, "Dear Sirs" and "Yours sincerely". As a result it is as easy to write a formal letter as it is to write a note to a friend. In addition, you don't have to find an envelope, write an address on it, find a stamp with the right denomination after you had to find out which denomination you need, don't forget to bring it to a mailbox or worse to a post office, the next of which is supposed to be very close to your place – but is it? – you know the game!

In E-mail, the equivalent for all this hassle is to push a button *Send*. Your message will be delivered in seconds, minutes or sometimes hours, to all addressees specified at once, and you can expect to get an answer from your recipients within hours to one or two days. I always answer E-mail the same day. I never do this with ordinary letters. E-mail combines the advantages of telephone calls (quick) and letters (no presence of recipient necessary).

There are some other services on the internet and on other networks (protocols) which are derivatives of E-mail: newsgroups, conferences, bulletin boards and mail lists:

1. Ordinary E-mail goes from one sender to one or more private mailboxes.
2. Conferences and newsgroups or bulletin boards are mail being sent to a mailbox which is accessible to everybody (public) or to members of a defined group.
3. Maillists are based on a software which resends all mail received to a mail list of subscribers (mail reflector).

To give you an impression of how useful electronic communication can be in professional communities, I quote an exchange of letters on Homeonet, an electronic conference on homeopathy on the IGC network (see Annex A of this paper).

Now I shall proceed from communication to information and publication.

Promises of the World Wide Web
The World Wide Web (WWW) is the most advanced method (turned into software) to present information on the Internet. It is basically text which may contain pictures and other graphic elements like a book or journal page, and, unlike a book page, also sound and video.

Then it may also contain hyperreferences, highlighted words (characters, sentences) which hide an invisible command to go some place. That place might be in the same document, in another document on the same server or somewhere on any WWW server in the world. Hyperreferences may be compared to literature references in scholarly texts. With one important difference: References tell you were to go, hyperreferences bring you there if you wish so.

Hyperreferences make hypertexts out of ordinary texts. Hypertexts are texts that are linked to each other, forming a network of "reference". This network is complemented (with an enormous amount of synergy!) by global networks of linked computers. The symbiosis of the two networks, the one consisting of "meaning" and the one consisting of satellites, copperwire and optical fibre, is going to change the way we write, read and work with texts. I can only mention some of the most important consequences:

1. By hyperreferences, text is structured according to interpretation-related criteria. That means, subjective, personal views of authors of hyperreferences are presented to users (who may in turn create hyperreferences themselves).
2. Formal structures like the beginning and the end of a text, sequences of chapters, addresses in directories, different computers on different locations, are not replaced but superimposed (rendered unimportant) by a content-related personal view.
3. There may be more than one personal view of a text; in fact, there may be as many views as there are ways of interpretation to a text. Looking at interpreters instead of interpretations, we see that a central perspective of someone who puts up a table of contents referring to the one formal structure of a text is supplemented by decentral perspectives of an indefinite number of people who supply their interpretations of a text.
4. Hyperreferencing makes the WWW at the same time millions of computers with billions of texts and one computer with one text.
5. Hyperreferencing also removes the border between a text I have written on my computer and a text outside somewhere on the Internet.
6. Independency and collaboration of workgroups becomes less of a contradiction than it used to be: Pooling resources and retaining full control over one's own material is easy in the publishing environment of the WWW. A "book" on the WWW can easily be made up of chapters, each of which may reside on different servers in different countries (say, e.g., Bethesda, MD., London, Copenhagen, Oslo, Stockholm, Montpelier, Zurich, Munich, Vienna).
7. Because hyperreferences are embedded in a context of sentences, their meaning may be defined to any extent of scholarly sophistication or spiritual depth. (Unlike a keyword which has no context! Also unlike a descriptor which has an external definition in a thesaurus; a definition, however, the user is usually unaware of!)

What services can Internet and other networks offer?
1. World wide electronic mail
2. Conferences, discussions, exchange of open letters on any conceivable subject with a worldwide audience
3. Exchange of manuscripts among members of workgroups – independent of their geographical location
4. Announcements of all kinds: events, publications, research, vacancies (everything a bulletin board does)
5. On-line searches in library catalogues, databases and other information sources

6. Electronic versions of journals and other publications which become available anywhere, anytime
7. Consulting, supervision: follow-up communication after personal education
8. Exchange of data among all the documentation and information services dealing with integrated medicine.

What services are actually being offered today on the Internet and other networks?

Today there are not too many groups in complementary medicine that use one or more of the above mentioned services for their communication needs. But this changes rapidly (see Literature and Annex B: *Sites to visit* in this paper). Wissensarchiv in Vienna tries to keep a list of interesting sites up to date (URL: http://www.magnet.at/Wissensarchiv/).

Outlook

Can scientific and therapeutic communities come closer together in cyberspace? Eli M. Noam argues in a very interesting article (Noam 1995: 247) that universities in their basic structure of locating

1. a library,
2. scholars,
3. and students

at one place will disappear, driven by the forces of

1. the explosive growth of published material,
2. specialization,
3. and the upcoming availability and relative cheapness of computer-based distant education.

If he is right, we can conclude that something like university structures for complementary medicine are unlikely to ever come into being. Universities, and with them, scientific communities, will develop into distributed networks of (electronically) published material and networks of people working with it and with each other.

Therapeutic and scientific communities in complementary medicine may develop to the same state "coming from the opposite direction." Distributed they are. Networks for collaboration and mutual information need to be developed. Given the technical means described above, that has never been easier.

References

Hancock, Lee
    1995   Internet/Bitnet Health Science Resource. Electronic Publication:
             URL: ftp://sura.net/pub/nic/medical.resources.2-23

Kovacs, Diane
    1995   Directory of Scholarly Electronic Conferences, 8th Rev. Electronic Publication: E-mail to:
             LISTSERV@KENTVM.KENT.EDU. Message: GET ACADLIST.README

Makulovich, John S.
    1994   Internet Resources on Alternative Medicine. Electronic Publication:
             URL: ftp://clark.net/pub/journalism/altmed.txt

Noam, Eli M.
    1995   "Electronics and the dim future of the university", in: *Science*, 270: 247-9.

Waltjen, Tobias; Schunder-Tatzber, Susanne.; Schwabl, Herbert.; Hoffmann-Dorninger, Renate
    1995   *Ganzheitsmedizin: Dokumentation, Information und Kommunikation. Bestandsaufnahme und Perspektiven aus österreichischer Sicht*, Facultas-Universitätsverlag: Wien.

Annex A: Example for therapeutic communication on Homeonet, an electronic conference on homeopathy on the IGC network[1]

<Eileen> on 22 Nov 1994:
I have a close friend who is at the end stage of stomach cancer. She has had most of her digestive tract removed but they never got all the cancer. It is now almost two weeks since she has had anything, food or liquid by mouth because to do so causes pain spasms that are unbearable. She discontinued the tube feedings because they also cause the pain. Right now she is fairly comfortable on morphine and says she will eat if she thinks it will feel right, she is not trying to starve herself on purpose. She is hydrated but obviously very weak. She is 5'11" tall and I estimate her weight to be close to 100 lbs.

Before she was this ill I had been taking her to one of the better known homeopaths in the Boston area because I was uncomfortable to treat a frein and because I thought the family would also be more comfortable. She was given Arsenicum 12c daily for the 1st month then increased to 200c, 1 dose with 12c daily to continue. She is now unable to keep any more appointments or make any phone calls so I said to keep taking the Ars. when she can. The rx still seems indicated to me so my question is do we keep up the daily low potency or raise it up. Some of my local homeopathic aquaintences say to give 3 doses of 1 or 10M with a 6x daily. I don't have much (any) expereince with terminal illness and have been afraid to give her higher potencies. I Have offered to supply a high dose when it is really near her time to die. I would appreciate all opinions and experiences while I go and reread whatever materials I can find of mine.
Eileen

<Rudi> on 22 Nov 1994:
Eileen,
I can sympathize with your situation and that of your friend.

If you think the remedy is indicated still, then I would gradually go up the scale to see if you can get some response. If you don't get any response to that, you might want to look at some smaller remedies that usuallly seem more indicated in severe pathology.

I have given cancer patients 1M at times without any severe risk of aggravation, but usually I would not go so high right away. You may just have to experiment with the range maybe even having to go up and then back down again.

You could also consider herbs, like Hydrastis, which is very good for the

---

1 Editors' note: These messages are presented as in the original therapeutic communication on the *Homeonet*. Consequently, the messages appear with all typing errors.

Stomach. You might also think of some intercurrent remedies, such as Cadmium sulph. which seems to work on many cancers. Viscum album is another herb which is often used in cancers generally.

In such cases, you could also give Carc. 200 or 1M with the other remedies. This is the time to try a "combination" as the case is severe and you need to try everything. There needs to be a method to the approach, but don' get caught up on the single remedy here if nothing seems to be working.
Rudi

<David> on 22 Nov 1994:
Give it based on the response. If the low potency lasts 2 hours give it every two hours. If it does nothing go up and try again. Unless you want to ehlp her to die now, i would avoid a high potency.
Best, david

<Rudi> on 23 Nov 1994:
Eileen,
Generally people say not to use the nosode for malignancies but a lot of the 19th and early 20th century cases in the books have been treated with Schirrum or Carcinosin. It can help if used judiciously, to unblock some pathways and let the well-indicated remdy work.

I have some Cadmium Sulph.. If you wish I could send a few doses down to you.

Keep up your efforts.
Rudi

<M.> on 23 Nov 1994:
The remedies that are curative in life are not necessarily the ones for dying. The similumum for life, may not be indicated for the transtion between worlds. As healers,we look the heal the body, as it is a vehicle for the soul. Our obligation is not to maintain it at all costs. If it is letting go, the case might look different. You need to ease the symptoms, make the person more confortable, look for remedies to facilitate the transition.
  m.

<Basil> on 23 Nov 1994:
Eileen:
The question I would ask is whether the Ars. is working?
   If not, then look for another remedy?
   You might want to review the remedy relationship tables (Gibson Miller).

Complementary remedies, to Ars., include: All-s., Carb-v., Natr-s., Phos., Pyrog., Thuja.

Remedies that follow well include: Aran., Arn., Apis, Ac-Fluor., Bar-c., Bell., Cact., Calc-phos., Cham., Chin., Cic., Ferr., Hep., Iod., Ipec., Kali-bic., Lach., Lyc., Merc., Nitr-S., Nux., Phos., Ran-sc., Sulph., Thuj., Verat.

You may be fortunate enough to see one of these remedies for the patient. Your review of the case will point you in the right direction.

If the patient was constitutionally Sulph., Ars. may have been the acute, and you may want to look closely at Sulph., Phos., Nux., and Acon.

In any case look at Phos., and Sulph.

Good luck

Basil

<Eileen> on 23 Nov 1994:

David and Rudi,

It was great to get your speedy responses and I am trying them. I slipped a bottle of hydrastis into her pocket today. I said she could take it in the feeding tube. The Ars. seems to work so I told her to repeat the 12c as needed and to try the 200 once in awhile. I don't have the cadmium sulph. but it sounds like a good idea. I am definately not committed to a single remedy at this point but I never took her case and have only the biased eye of a friend. It has also been suggested to use an intercurrent nosode and this is where the lack of case taking is a problem. I thought Carc. wasn't supposed to be good for malignancies. What about Ornithogalum which is the rx I wanted to give before the surgery in fact even before the diagnosis because it covered the pain so well?

Many thanks,

Eileen

<Greg> on 23 Nov 1994:

Hi Eileen,

It sounds like a tough situation.

I have doubts about Ars. being the simillimum. If it were correct, it seems that the pt would have shown SOME signs of ameloration, ey? I would re-take the case (and post it here if you want) and perhaps try another remedy in low daily doses, based on her response. 200-c or higher can cause an agg. — there is always this risk, especially in weak patients, and especially if repeated daily. I prefer 12-c daily myself, in such cases.

This is the time to pull out the stops and try other modalities but don't throw them at her, prescribe consciously, based on the patients symptoms and response.

I have had loved ones die in my arms before, two-timed by the ravages of disease and the abuse of heroic medicine. It made me hate allopathy but later embrace homeopathy. The thing I have learned is to concentrate my focus on easing their pain and doing it in such a way that they retain as much dignity as possible.

"Two things (of importance) happen, one in the beginning, and one at the end"
Greg

<Ken> on 27 Nov 1994:
Eileen:
I wish I could comment on a remedy selection. There are those wiser than many who have responded to your queries. All I can offer you is a word of support. Caring for a dying friend or loved one is a heart rending task.

Take care of yourself. It sounds trite, but try to preceive what the person wants. Continued life or transition.

Regardless, I'm proud of you for trying to help.
Be well.
Ken

<Eileen> on 27 Nov 1994:
Basil, <m>,and Rudi,
I have read all your suggestions and kind words and and picking and choosing what makes sense to me from all you have offered. I plan to study all the rx you suggested Basil. I will let everyone know how I decide to proceed. A few answers for now. Yes the arsenicum is working. The days she takes it she definately has more energy. She is also now taking essiac tea which she discovered herself when looking for alternatives to chemo.

I definately feel this is not the time for only the one correct rx and plan to try a couple with a nososde inter- spersed. The good news is that she is doing better now so I think her vital force will respond well to the remedies. A few days ago I would not have believed what I saw today was possible. She has begun eating again (real food) after a month of not taking anything by mouth including water. Now she is actually hungry and food is going down well with no spasms. When I arrived today to visit she was making turkey soup from he leftover turkey! In all the talk about rx I have never mentioned that I thinkARs was probably always her "constitutional" Thank you all for all the helpful suggestions. I'll keep you posted.
Eileen

<Eileen> on 28 Nov 1994:
KEN,
Thanks for your support. So far the choice is to continue the fight.
   Eileen

Annex B: Internet Sites to Visit (examples; updated February 1996)

Search Engines
Altavista. URL: http://www.altavista.digital.com/
Excite. URL: http://www.excite.com/
Yahoo. URL: http://www.yahoo.com/Health/Medicine/

in German language
Ärztewoche Online, Wien. URL: http://www.aerztewoche.co.at/aerztewoche/

Ganzheitsmedizin Online, Wien. URL: http://www.magnet.at/Wissenarchiv/

Gesundheitsinformationsnetz, Universität Innsbruck.
URL: http://info.uibk.ac.at/gin/

Patienteninformationssystem, FU Berlin.
URL: http://www.ukbf.fuberlin.de/UKBF/NHK/d_pi.htm (also in English)

in English language
Courses on Alternative Therapies Taught At Conventional U.S. Medical Schools. URL: http://www.amrta.org/~amrta/courses.html

CPMCnet: Rosenthal Center.
URL: http://cpmcnet.columbia.edu/dept/rosenthal/guide.html

Homeopathic Web Server, Cambridge. URL: http://www.dungeon.com/home/cam/homeo.html

IGC (Institute for Global Communication)
URL: gopher://gopher.igc.apc.org/11/health

International Network for Research on Alternative Therapies (INRAT), Copenhagen. URL: http://inet.uni-c.dk/~inrathj

Part V

Dialogues and Politics

"So-called Alternative Treatment"

On the medical profession's views on quackery and alternative medicine in Sweden

by Motzi Eklöf

I would like to give you the Swedish version of a story that may be recognizable in other countries. It concerns the fact that the borderline between the authorized and the non-authorized health care sector has changed in recent years, as some previous alternative therapists now have the opportunity to get a governmental licence. This was decided against the will of the organized medical profession. There are also obvious differences between the official standpoint of the medical profession and the opinion of practising physicians concerning alternative medicine.

In the years 1986 to 1989 I worked for the Swedish Committee on Alternative Medicine, which was set up by the Swedish government. The proposals from the Committee, presented in 1989, were then circulated for consideration amongst the parties concerned. I also compiled their answers for the Ministry of Health and Social Affairs. Doing this work, I gained insight into the views of the organized medical profession concerning alternative medicine. By the organized profession I mean the union, the Swedish Medical Association (*Sveriges läkarförbund*), and the scientific organization, the Swedish Society of Medicine (*Svenska Läkaresällskapet*). Alternative medicine was looked upon as a phenomenon, the existence of which unfortunately had to be accepted – with reference to historical traditions and popular belief – but whose forms and contents ought to be restricted and controlled (Alternativmedicinkommittén/AMK/ 1989a: 222-23; Läkartidningen/LT/ 1990: 2469). I will quote a sentence from the Medical Association's answer to the proposals presented by the Committee, dated 1989 (all quotations translated):

> "There can (. . .) hardly be any reason to encourage the individual to avail himself of alternative treatment, as there – in spite of efforts – has not in any case been demonstrated any positive effect of such treatment" (Sveriges läkarförbund 1989).

I find a statement like that interesting, from different perspectives.

I am presently researching the history of the medical profession's discourse and strategies concerning alternative medicine in Sweden during this century. The history of alternative medicine is also the history of what previously has been called 'quackery'. I will start with a short review of the legal-legislative proceedings regarding quackery and alternative medicine during the 20th century and then go on to say something about the opinions on the topic expressed by the medical profession. I will put these opinions in relation to some studies done on ordinary practising physicians' attitudes towards alternative medicine.

The Quackery Laws in Sweden

During the 17th century the medical profession was still quite small in number. In 1688 the Swedish Collegium Medicum, founded some years earlier, granted the medical profession the exclusive right to practise the art of medicine as well as the right to supervise and restrain quackery (Wistrand 1857). Towards the end of the 19th century the medical profession demanded a more modern law concerning quackery. The prevailing Act was considered too permissive. It set, e.g., fines as low as 12 crowns and 50 öre, which was not considered a sufficient deterrent for the flourishing business of selling patent medicines and other forms of quackery (Norgren 1912: 96-97).

In 1915 a new law was instituted, regulating the authorization in the field of medicine (Svensk författningssamling/SFS/ 1916). The new Act turned out to be a disappointment to the medical profession. It prohibited everyone except authorized doctors from practising the art of medicine when payment was involved, but offenders could only be prosecuted if their treatment endangered the patient's life or health. The intention behind the new Act was to provide for intervention against the activities of nostrum-mongers, homeopaths and other professional quacks, but not to impede the activities of the local folk healers in the countryside, where authorized doctors were rare.

With the passing of this Act the doctors actually lost their monopoly. In the text of the Act the word quackery was not used. In an article in the Swedish Medical Journal the Act was later described as the decriminalization of quackery (Haglund 1936: 1763-64).

A governmental investigation in the 1950s resulted in a new law against quackery which was passed in 1960 (Kvacksalveriutredningen 1956; SFS 1961). According to this law, laymen are free to practise the art of medicine with certain specified exceptions. They are not, e.g., allowed to treat pregnant women or children under 8, nor certain conditions like cancer; also certain methods of treatment are prohibited. The law contains the possibility of imposing punishment for quackery that endangers a person's life or health. This Act is still valid with some minor amendments.

In 1989 the Committee on Alternative Medicine presented a proposal for a new law concerning the practice of alternative medicine, but this proposal has not (yet) resulted in a new law (AMK 1989a).

Inside and Outside Authorized Health Care

The borderline has changed between quackery and alternative medicine on the one hand, and authorized health care on the other.

According to the governmental investigation in the 50s, the category of quacks at that time included homeopaths, chiropractors, osteopaths (although there was only one in Sweden), naturopaths, sellers of patent medicines, traditional folk-healers etc. It also included occupational groups such as psychoanalysts and speech therapists (Kvacksalveriutredningen 1956: 86). In the middle of the 80s, when I worked for the new governmental investigation, I counted about 200 different types of alternative treatment (AMK 1989b). By that time psychologists and traditional psychotherapists had obtained governmental authorization and were not considered to be "alternative" any longer.

Although the old quackery law from 1960 is still valid, some proposals made by the Committee have actually been effectuated. One is that in 1989 Doctors of Chiropractic were given the opportunity to get governmental authorization. In 1994 the parliament decided that the time had come for authorization of Doctors of Naprapathy. The entry of these new occupational groups into the health services was decided against the will of the medical profession.

The arguments expressed by the organized medical profession against the proposal for authorization of chiropractors were mainly three:

1. There has not been shown any positive effect of manipulation of the spine to compensate for the risks of such treatment.
2. Proper education in this discipline is not available in Sweden. Therefore, it is not possible to control and influence such education.
3. There are enough authorized physicians and physiotherapists who can provide adequate treatment. Therefore, there is no use for chiropractors (AMK 1987: 80-82; LT 1987a: 1103).

The concepts of quackery and alternative medicine can either be a more or less neutral denomination of non-authorized treatments, or a more normative description of the character of therapies quite different from conventional scientific biomedicine. During the first half of the century, these two meanings of the concept of quackery overlapped. What complicates the use of the term alternative medicine today is that therapies such as chiropractic and naprapathy, earlier considered to be "alternative," and by the medical profession still considered to be "alternative," now have been accepted in authorized health care.

The Swedish Medical Journal

I have gone through the Medical Journal (*Läkartidningen*), published by the Medical Association, from its start in 1904 until 1994. The articles in the journal dealing with quackery and alternative medicine are in the index listed under mainly three keywords. Up to the 1970s the keyword is Quackery, from 1973 to 1988 it is Therapeutic Cults. The term therapeutic cults is used exclusively in the index, never in the articles themselves. In 1986 the term Alternative Medicine appears as a separate keyword. These keywords succeed each other and there are often cross-references between them.

An example from the journal's index of 1988: here an article about naprapathy is not listed under the word Naprapathy in the index – it is referred to Quackery. Naprapathy is otherwise in the 1970s and 1980s listed directly under Therapeutic Cults, together with chiropractic and other unorthodox treatment methods.

The term quackery suggests ignorance, incompetence, superstitious beliefs, fraud – in any case something far removed from science and medical professionalism. And whatever first associations you get when you hear the term therapeutic cult, they surely have a negative ring. A cult is described as a common worship of a certain god or other holy phenomenon practised in ceremonial acts, especially in so-called primitive religions (Norstedt 1985). If this – with the addition of the meaning of the word therapeutic – is taken to be the Medical Journal's conception of chiropractic and naprapathy not very long ago, it is not surprising that the medical profession is against the idea of integrating practitioners of these disciplines into regular health care.

A survey through all first-page articles and editorials in the Medical Journal concerning unconventional treatment methods shows that during the past 90-year period quackery has turned into alternative medicine, patent or humbug medicines have been replaced by natural remedies, but the difference from the viewpoint of the medical profession seems to be none or little.[1] The descriptions

---

[1] These articles reveal the more official standpoint of the profession; other articles and contributions in the journal may show other opinions and attitudes.

of quackery and its consequences, the arguments against quackery and measures considered desirable to be taken against it by the medical profession itself and the authorities have not changed very much. There have, though, been changes concerning the descriptions of the patients going to quacks: by and by the descriptions have become less disrespectful. On the other hand, the disappointment with the politicians and the authorities in the health care field has become more clearly expressed.

Quackery has always been described as a growing problem – a cause for concern in itself – and a market changing in character in an alarming way: from local folk healing to professional "geschäft"-making.

Especially during the first half of the century quackery was described as falsifications, ignorance, authoritarian doctrines of faith, fraud, mysticism, nonsense, superstition etc. In 1912 the quacks themselves are described as *"Hocuspocus-makers: preachers and storekeepers, former tailors and shoemakers, travelling salesmen, workmen, medical orderlies, hospital hands – may the Good Lord have mercy on the whole bunch of them!"* (Norgren 1912: 87). In later years the vocabulary becomes less forceful, but there is still talk about "geschäft", fortune hunters making money on people's credulity, and dubious and hazardous activities; the latter applies to chiropractors as late as 1987 (LT 1987a: 1104).

People consulting quacks, the patients, are in the early years of the century described as stupid, attracted to mysticism and religion, turning against the natural sciences, unfavourably disposed towards the rational and scientific. They are said to be poor foolish victims etc. In 1906, for instance, patients are described as *"suggestible neurotics and in slighter degree psychologically abnormal . . . a clientele that easier than others is influenced by such therapy; nervous, hysterical, neurasthenic as well as people with some symptomatic trash diagnoses like hiccup"* (Santesson 1906: 246). Today, the patients are not described in such a contemptuous manner, but the word "credulous" is still used (LT 1989: 3523).

When it comes to the treatment of disease, it is said that the patients do not suffer from real diseases, or that they do have serious diseases which the quacks cannot diagnose, much less treat adequately. In the case of the quacks giving treatment, it is called symptom-oriented or dangerous. Whenever the treatment leads to recovery, it is explained as illusory, due to suggestion (Santesson 1906: 245-46, Norgren 1912: 94). Today the main argument against alternative medicine is that it has no real effects, that there is no scientific proof of the efficacy of the methods or remedies (Svenska LT 1964: 2418-20, LT 1974: 1045, 1987a: 1103). Even if the treatment given by a quack should be harmless in itself, it is said that the danger with quackery and alternative medicine is that it may delay, neglect or interrupt the competent, adequate, rational, modern and scientific medicine (e.g., Santesson 1906: 245, LT 1988: 4007).

The term alternative medicine is used only reluctantly by the medical profession. When it appears in the editorials of the Medical Journal it is usually put within quotation-marks or preceded by the expression "so-called". I suppose that the dislike of this new concept indicates the author's opinion that alternative medicine is neither a real alternative nor a real treatment.

The medical profession has always been careful to emphasize that it represents the interests of the patients and of society and that its proposals for measures against quackery are *not* a matter of professional egoism. It is said that *"The quality of medical care is more important than such narrow interests."* And:

> "The critical comments by the Medical Association against authorization of chiropractors come (. . .) above all from its concern about the safety of medical care and the reputation of medical science" (LT 1987b: 2831).

What should be done, then, to reduce the harmful effects of quackery and alternative medicine? Restrictive legislation, controlled marketing and advertising, popular education in health matters, keeping medicine clean from alternative methods, unbiased research and a better official health care – these are the measures proposed, with various intensity (e.g., Santesson 1906: 247-48, Norgren 1912: 96-97, LT 1979: 3258). Previously, also information about the nature of quackery was recommended. This is no longer the case. Gone are the long articles in the Medical Journal on homeopathy humbug medicines as published at the beginning of the century.

Seen from the perspective of the medical profession, the political decisions seldom have gone its way (even if others see it differently). Editorials in the Medical Journal in the last decades talk about measures being taken *"under political pressure"* (LT 1975: 4579) and about *"political considerations (that) have ruled out the demands for safety"* (LT 1980: 2655), and it is said that the proposal to authorize chiropractors has been worked out *"on order from the Ministry of Health and Social Affairs"* (LT 1987c: 3792).

Different Views on Alternative Medicine within the Medical Profession

This was the official, dissociative standpoint of the medical profession towards alternative medicine.

What practising doctors actually *do* is quite another thing. There have always been doctors using unconventional methods or cooperating with unauthorized healers. In Sweden today there is a Physicians Group for Anthroposophical Medicine (*Läkarföreningen för Antroposofiskt Orienterad Medicin*) as well as an Association for Biological Medicine (*Svenska Läkares Förening för Biologisk Medicin*). There are physicians that have long been cooperating with chiropractors and naprapaths. There are physicians that are using homeopathic remedies, although homeopathy in Sweden is not considered to be in accordance with "scientific knowledge and proven experience", which is required of the methods used by medical doctors according to their instructions (Hälso- och sjukvårdslagen 1994). The laws regulating the pharmaceutical area have now been harmonized with the legislation of other countries in the European Union, and homeopathic as well as anthroposophical remedies are integrated in the new law of 1993.

In 1988 and 1990 two studies were conducted which attempted to reveal Swedish physician's attitudes towards and experiences of alternative medicine. The first study consisted of a sample of one-tenth of Swedish physicians, of whom 65% completed the questionnaire (Elmberg & Eriksson 1988). The second study encompassed both conventional physicians and physicians who were members of the mentioned associations for unconventional medicine (Lynöe & Svensson 1992). Some of the results from these studies are especially interesting when put in relation to the medical profession's official views on alternative medicine.

According to the first study, about 2% of the physicians chose to define alternative medicine with words like "geschäft," "false doctrines" etc. 17% defined the term as badly or not documented medicine. One-third of the physicians defined alternative medicine as being unconventional medicine, not established medicine etc. The more neutral definitions were in the majority.

The physicians were also asked how much they knew about different alternative methods of treatment. Concerning chiropractic, 2% said it was a harmful method; 66% thought it to be effective. Naprapathy was thought to be effective by 28%; 1% thought it was harmful; the method was unknown to 38% of the physicians. Not 1% of the physicians stated that chiropractic or naprapathy was an ineffective method. Questioned about whether Doctors of Chiropractic should get governmental authorization, more than half agreed, whereas one-third disagreed.

The other study mentioned compared the attitudes towards different alternative methods of treatment between conventional and unconventional physicians. Concerning manual therapy, 47% of the conventional physicians were positive, in comparison to about 77% of the unconventional ones.

Some Comments

The medical profession in itself has changed during this century and become more heterogeneous. Also the role of the medical profession in the total health care sector has changed, as well as the relation between the medical profession and the state. During the 20th century the medical profession in Sweden has had less influence on the shaping of the health care system than maybe could be expected, due to different circumstances (Bjurulf & Swahn 1980, Garpenby 1989, Ito 1980, Hamel 1985). Alternative medicine is another field where the development has taken a course not appreciated by the medical profession.

Biomedicine and the medical profession are no longer considered to have the answer to all health problems. Even if the organized medical profession officially will not recognize any positive effects of alternative treatment, other persons and institutions obviously do, including quite a number of ordinary physicians. Politicians and authorities in the health care field also take into consideration other things than scientific biomedical knowledge when planning for future health care. Seen from the perspective of the medical profession, the state was at the beginning of the century at least a theoretical confederate in the struggle against quackery – now it seems to be another enemy, hard to defeat.

Where alternative medicine is concerned, the organized medical profession seems to have talked itself into a position where there is no return without the cracking of the whole idea of scientific medicine as the foundation for authorized health care. Trying to communicate about alternative therapies this official way is hard; the layers of rhetoric formed during decades and centuries are deep. Still, it is the medical profession's top representatives who are sitting on governmental committees concerning alternative medicine, delivering comments on proposals etc. The communication problem between physicians and alternative therapists, between medical and other researchers concerning for instance evaluation of treatment effects, has to be solved on another, less official and rhetorical level.

References

Alternativmedicinkommittén
1987   *Legitimation för vissa Kiropraktorer. Delbetänkande av Alternativmedicinkommittén*, Statens Offentliga Utredningar 1987: 12, Allmänna förlaget: Stockholm.

1989a   *Alternativ Medicin 1. Huvudbetänkande från Aternativmedicinkommittén*, Statens Offentliga Utredningar 1989: 60, Allmänna Förlaget: Stockholm.

1989b   *Alternativ Medicin 3. Alternativa Terapier i Sverige – en Kartläggning*, Statens Offentliga Utredningar 1989: 62, Allmänna förlaget: Stockholm.

Bjurulf, Bo & Swahn, Urban
1980   "Health Policy Proposals and What Happened to Them: Sampling the Twentieth-century Record", in: Arnold J. Heidenheimer & Nils Elvander (eds.): *The Shaping of the Swedish Health System*, Croom Helm: London.

Elmberg, Birgitta & Eriksson, Carl-Gunnar
1990   "Läkarkåren och alternativmedicinen", in: *Socialmedicinsk tidskrift*, 67(9-10): 510-515.

Garpenby, Peter
1989   *The State and the Medical Profession. A Cross-National Comparison of the Health Policy Arena in the United Kingdom and Sweden 1945-1985*, (Diss.), Linköping Studies in Arts and Science 39, Department of Health and Society: Linköping.

Haglund, Patrik
1936   "Aktuella synpunkter på kvacksalverifrågan", in: *Svenska Läkartidningen*, 33(49): 1761-75.

Hamel, Matthew
1985   "Sveriges läkarförbund och utvecklingen av sjukvårdssystemet", in: *Socialmedicinsk tidskrift*, 62(2-3): 127-30.

Hälso- och Sjukvårdslagen
1994   "Allmän läkarinstruktion (1963: 341; ändr. senast 1992: 962)", in: Jan Sahlin (ed.): *Hälso- och sjukvårdslagen med kommentarer*, 4th ed, Fritzes: Stockholm.

Ito, Hirobumi
1980   "Health Insurance and Medical Services in Sweden and Denmark 1850-1950", in: Arnold J. Heidenheimer & Nils Elvander (eds.): *The Shaping of the Swedish Health System*, Croom Helm: London.

Kvacksalveriutredningen
1956   *Lag om Rätt att Utöva Läkekonsten. Förslag avgivet av Kvacksalveriutredningen*. Statens offentliga utredningar 1956: 29, Stockholm.

Lynöe, Niels & Svensson, Tomas
1992   "Physicians and Alternative Medicine – An Investigation of Attitudes and Practice", in: *Scandinavian Journal of Social Medicine*, 20: 55-60.

Läkartidningen editorials
1974   "Den 'nya' akupunkturen", in: *Läkartidningen*, 71(11): 1045.

1975   "Den heliga kon", in: *Läkartidningen*, 72(47): 4579-80.

1980   "Dubbelmoral!", in: *Läkartidningen*, 77(32-33): 2655.

1987a   "Tillsyn – inte legitimation!", in: *Läkartidningen*, 84(14): 1103-04.

1987b   "Vårdpengar till alternativen?", in: *Läkartidningen*, 84(37): 2831.

1987c   "Vem försvarar säkerheten nu?", in: *Läkartidningen*, 84(46): 3791-92.

1989   "Halvmesyr om alternativen", in: *Läkartidningen*, 86(42): 3523.

1990   "Skydda konsumenterna!", in: *Läkartidningen*, 87(32-22): 2469.

Norgren, C. Arvid
1912   "Homöopatien i Sverige och dess utöfvare", in: *Allmänna Svenska Läkartidningen*, 9(6): 81-97.

Norstedt
1985   *Norstedts Uppslagsbok: Illustrerad Encyklopedi i ett Band*, 3rd print 1987, Norstedt: Stockholm.

Santesson, C. G.
1906   "Några ord om homöopatien", in: *Allmänna Svenska Läkartidningen*, 3(15 and 16): 225-33 and 241-48.

Svensk Författningssamling
1916   "Lag (1915: 362) om Behörighet att Utöva Läkekonsten", in: *Svensk Författningssamling för 1915, del I*, P. A. Norstedt & Söner: Stockholm.

1961   "Lag (1960: 409) om Förbud i vissa Fall mot Verksamhet på Hälso- och Sjukvårdens Område", in: *Svensk Författningssamling för 1960, del II*, P. A. Norstedt & Sönder: Stockholm.

Svenska läkartidningen
1964   "Disciplinnämnden och THX" (ed.), in: *Svenska läkartidningen*, 61: 2418-20.

Sveriges läkarförbund
1989   Unpublished *remissyttrande* concerning SOU 1989: 60, Reg no S 4895/89, Ministry of Health and Social Affairs: Stockholm.

Wistrand, Hilarion A.
1857   "K. M:ts Medicinal-ordningar af år 1688, eller Privilegier som K. M:t förunnat Coll. Medicum", in: Hilarion A. Wistrand: *Författningar Angående Medicinal-väsendet i Sverige*, P. A. Norstedt & Söner: Stockholm.

The Story of a Dialogue Group between Practitioners of Alternative (Traditional) Medicine and Modern (Western) Medicine in Norway

by Vigdis Moe Christie

A dialogue group consisting of alternative practitioners as well as doctors and nurses was started in Oslo in 1989.[1] The reasons for starting this group were manifold; I will point to three of them:

1. Many patients in Norway, as well as in many other countries, consult ordinary doctors as well as alternative health practitioners. Most patients do not exclude one or the other. In Norway today we think that is the case for 1/3 of the population. Among people who are seriously ill about 50% go to see alternative practitioners (Christie 1991b).

It is important to remember that consulting an alternative practitioner in Norway is not refunded by the official health system (except for seeing a chiropractor, then you can get a very small amount repaid providing you can find a doctor willing to write a requisition).

One of the reasons so many patients consult both doctors and alternative practitioners may result from the phenomenon that doctors diagnose and treat diseases as they define them from a biomedical point of view. The patients, however, are concerned with their own particular experience of their illnesses. Eisenberg and others have demonstrated how differences in the doctors' and patients' explanatory models may lead to communication problems in the clinical setting (Eisenberg 1977, Kleinman, Eisenberg and Good 1978, Kleinman 1980, Sachs 1983 and Malterud 1987).

2. In Norway most practitioners of these two professions never meet professionally, unless it is as debaters in scientific and professional journals. They receive information about each other through newspaper headlines, when something bad has happened, involving one or the other, through the coloured press, or through discontented patients who have been unsuccessfully treated by the other part. In

---

[1] An article about this dialogue group has been printed in *Social Science and Medicine* (Christie 1991).

these ways, physicians and alternative practitioners get an insufficient and biased report on one another's practices, as well as an unrealistic and distorted picture of one another. These are all situations that create antagonism and suspicion rather than mutual respect and cooperation. Mahler formulated it like this back in 1977, though it holds equally true for the situation in Norway today:

> "For too long, traditional and modern medicine have followed their own separate paths in mutual antipathy. But their aims are surely identical: the improvement of human health and, hence, improvement of the quality of life."

Ursula Sharma (1990) writes:

> "The crucial issue at present is how communication between the orthodox and nonorthodox health care professionals can be coordinated at the local level."

The lack of openness which modern medicine shows vis-a-vis alternative medicine in industrialized countries is probably related precisely to these countries' high level of industrialization. Technical solutions based on modern science and mass production have gained what Ivan Illich (1974) calls radical monopoly. It is a solution which through its seeming success is pushing all other alternatives aside. This is also in accordance with Eisenberg (1977), who writes that models "...*are ways of constructing reality, of imposing meaning on the chaos of the phenomenal world,*" and "*once in place, models act to generate their own verification by excluding phenomena outside the frame of reference the user employs.*"

3. If patients know that both parties respect one another, even though they might disagree on many questions, then many, or maybe most of the patients, would dare admit that they used both types of practitioners. Otherwise many patients conceal this. Many of my informants said they even *are afraid* that their physicians may learn of it. They feel that this dishonesty in a way spoils the trust between doctor and patient.

The picture is nearly as bad as this:

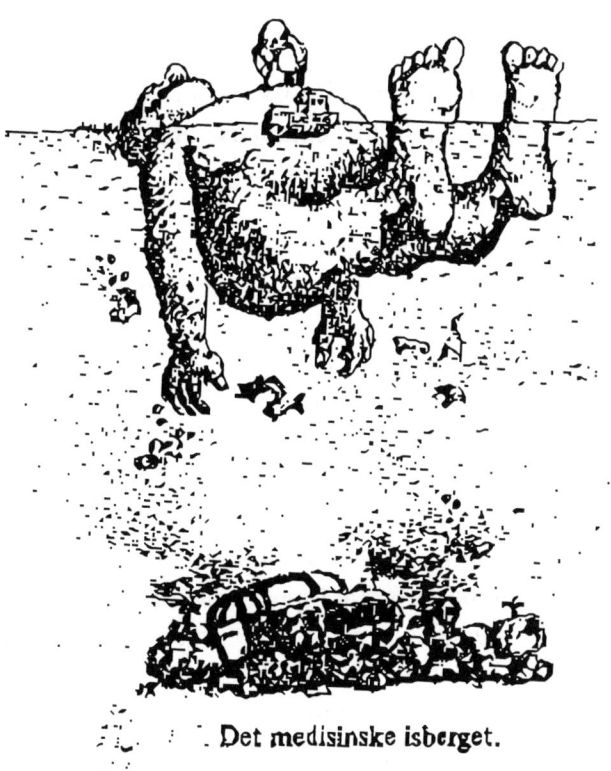

. Det medisinske isberget.

Figure 1: This picture shows the large number of patients who go to see alternative practitioners. The doctor only knows about those of his patients above the surface.

When I first went to one of the health centres in Oslo and put forward my plans for starting a dialogue group, they were negatively disposed, because they had – they told me – interviewed a number of their patients seven years earlier about different health questions. Only a little more than 10% of the patients admitted that they had consulted an alternative practitioner at least once. I said:

> "I do not think you then got honest answers. If you tell the patients that you are considering to start a dialogue group with some alternative practitioners, then your patients will more likely feel free to talk about their use of alternatives."

The three doctors at the health centre followed my proposal
To their astonishment 58 (51%) of the 114 patients they asked had been consulting alternative practitioners. Fifty-one (45%) mentioned such contact within their immediate family circle. As many as 98 (86%) expressed a positive attitude towards alternative practitioners. The general use of alternative practitioners had grown during these seven years, not least in the Oslo area, but not to such a high degree, not from 10 to 51%.

After this experience the dialogue group was started in January 1989. We went on with regular meetings for about five years. The last one and a half years we have had a pause.

One of the general practitioners at the health centre, Edwin Sandberg, was together with myself the co-initiator of the dialogue group. He died of leukemia in 1993. Edwin Sandberg had already had positive experiences from cooperating with a "United Health Group" as part of his work in primary health care in Botswana.

In some developing countries "health committees" have been established to create a dialogue between the different types of health professionals. In this way traditional practitioners are seen as a resource group in the primary health care system. In industrialized countries little of this seems to have been done so far.

Cooperation between two quite different medical systems is, of course, difficult when their language, concepts and practice vary widely (Fulder 1987, Ingstad 1989).

It seems reasonable to us, living in the Western world, that health committees should be established in developing countries. But we do not find the need for them so pressing in industrialized countries. It is obvious that alternative medicine in Scandinavia is not the same as traditional medicine in Third World countries. The idea, however, of integrating the best aspects of these two medical systems nonetheless seems valid.

The dialogue group
Our group consisted of *nine persons*. Three practised alternative medicine in the form of acupuncture, homeopathy and chiropractic. Three others were general practitioners and two were nurses, all five working at the same health centre. The ninth member, myself, a social scientist, was a participant observer, a patient, a coordinator as well as a "diplomat".

Our first aim was to find alternative practitioners working in the same area where the health centre was located. Only one was found, a chiropractor. The acupuncturist as well as the homeopath had their practices not too far away.

Homeopathy, chiropractic and acupuncture, which we concentrated on, are the most common in use, at least in the Oslo area. It might also have been conceivable, of course, to have included representatives from other alternative medical professions as well as from more old-fashioned forms of what we can call "traditional" Norwegian practitioners, e.g., healers. But we abstained from that idea. Representatives of these forms were few and far between, especially in this area. At the same time their methods were even less understood. A considerable amount of work would have to be done before they could be included in a system productive of mutual understanding. Besides, having too many different practitioners could prove difficult, we were afraid. Seen in retrospect, it was difficult enough.

The meetings of the dialogue group
In the beginning the group met every month for two to three hours in the evening. At each meeting, one specific disease fairly common in the practices of the group members was discussed. Each practitioner explained what she or he would do with a patient suffering from this disease. For example, patients with whiplash injuries were discussed at several meetings. While talking about these patients, and how it might be possible to better help them, the peculiarities of the respective fields come up. It was possible in this way to get a much more concrete discussion of each individual case. Programmatic declarations nearly never appeared; instead, a situation was created where different types of "helpers" discussed in detail how they would handle the case to the maximum benefit of the patient.

A great amount of agreement prevailed among the members of the group since they all focused on the patient. There have been discussions both of treatment and of each patient's social and psychological circumstances (Karoliussen 1988). It seems that not only the alternative practitioners but the doctors as well, have the habit of listening to the patient and taking time during the consultation to let the patient talk when necessary. This is in contrast to the impression many patients have and also express about doctors (Christie 1987, Bannerman, Burton and Ch'en 1983). Helman (1984) writes:

> "The 'model' of modern medicine is mainly directed towards discovering, and quantifying physio-chemical information about the patient, rather than less measurable social and emotional factors."

As Kleinman (1980) writes, the Western doctor's view of clinical reality "... *assumes that biologic concerns are more basic, 'real', clinically significant, and interesting than psychological and sociocultural issues."*

Because the modern health personnel in our dialogue group worked as employees at a municipal health centre, they were probably able to spend more time with each patient than is often the case for doctors working in private practices or in hospitals.

Some might argue that their verbal assertions stem from their wish to present themselves in a certain light in this special situation (Goffman 1959). This may be the reason they put such strong emphasis on patient management. But this does not seem to be the case. They are all quite secure and of high standing in their professions. They meet because of their common role of being those who can help patients. The presence of a social scientist seems to have strengthened the common identification of the others as possessing skills for treating sick and disabled people and their illnesses (Mills 1967).

The first two years we were only to a very small extent occupied with the principles or theories of the different systems. I purposely hindered that, and we concentrated our attention on special diseases that all the practitioners found hard to cure, or even help the patients with.

Later in the career of the group we increasingly started to discuss the principles behind the different therapies. This, I must confess, has often been difficult. For nurses or physicians, with the training they have, it is not easy to understand how the homeopathic medicine works, or to hear about the meridians running through our bodies that are so essential for the acupuncturist. Health personel have never been taught during their training that such meridians even existed.

I remember once when the chiropractor was speaking of the importance of the spine, or spinal column, he mentioned that nearly all the persons present were sitting in a position in their chairs that harmed their spines. One of the doctors, who was more or less lying in his little spindleback chair, took exception to this remark, or maybe he took it as a correction, I do not know. In any case, it came to a dispute. The chiropractor felt he knew the most about the spine since it had been his focus during his five years of training, not to mention his 15 years of practice. The doctor was equally insistent on his own behalf. I managed to calm them down by cracking a joke. But mostly, happily enough, the atmosphere in the group has been one of trust and frankness as well as curiosity.

The last years of our meetings, the practitioners started to collaborate in the treatment of some of their patients. There, the physicians could see the effect of the alternative treatment on their own patients that they knew very well. In this way they experienced what other professionals might be able to achieve, even if it was hard to understand the principles behind the practice.

Let me give some examples: The very first patient, who was recommended by her doctor working at the centre to see an alternative practitioner, was a lady who had been suffering from migraine or headache for about 40 years. The only help she had gotten was pain-killing tablets. The chiropractor was able to help her with her pains. Later, other patients with migraine followed.

The chiropractor said he wanted to get whiplash patients in the first three weeks after the accident, because it then would be more likely he could prevent, for example, headaches. I do not think this has been tried yet in our group.

Another patient who was discussed in the group, was an eleven year old boy who had been suffering from asthma for some years. They had known him and his family at the health centre since he was a tiny baby. He had always been a happy and healthy child. The asthma had suddenly appeared. They felt it could not be psychosomatic. The chiropractor said it might come from a defect in his spine. *"My God, not everything can be the result of a spine defect,"* exclaimed one of the nurses. The doctors discussed it for some weeks, and at last the boy went to see the chiropractor. He was actually helped. For the people working at the health centre, who had seen him for a long time suffering badly from asthma, it was nearly unbelievable. But even then it took some time before other patients with asthma followed.

The last patient I will mention here was a woman, 35 years of age. She had chronic cystitis (infection of the urinary tract). She had also had pyelitis (inflammation of the renal pelvis). She had been taking sulfa-preparations. She was helped by the homeopath, and her troubles did not reappear. The homeopath had also recommended that she cut down on sugar in her diet; it would be a help in avoiding getting the infection back. Some other patients with the same trouble were then recommended to the homeopath.

After having met nearly every month for several years, we went down to about five to six meetings a year. The last 1 1/2 years we have had a pause because everything was working fine. The involved parts knew each other so well, they could phone each other when they had something to discuss. It is, of course, much easier for a doctor to suggest to one of his patients to go see an alternative practitioner when he knows the practitioner personally, knows he has a good education and is a competent as well as an agreeable person.

But during the last year the interaction between the health centre and the alternative practitioners has dried out. It is as if they needed the meetings we had to remember that there can be other solutions to the troubles patients experience than the ones they once were trained to deal with. Another reason is that Edwin Sandberg has died. He was the most enthusiastic of the staff at the health centre about this cooperation. The dialogue group is not what it was any longer. We may have to start all over again with the old health centre. Our original plan was to meet again this winter. I have also been urged to start new groups elsewhere in Oslo.

Since we started this group several joint practices with physicians and alternative practitioners have appeared, especially in the bigger cities in Norway. But the main difference is that they, as far as I know, consist of physicians and alternative practitioners who were on speaking terms with one another, and who respected each other *before* they started their office fellowship.

References

Bannerman, R. H., Burton, J. and Ch'en Wen-Chieh (eds.)
    1983   *Traditional Medicine and Health Care Coverage. A Reader for Health Administrators and Practitioners*, World Health Organization: Geneva.

Christie, Vigdis Moe
    1987   "Skolemedisinen som grobunn for den alternative medisin" (Conventional medicine as a fertile soil for alternative medicine), in: *Nordisk Medisin*, 102: 318-319.

    1991   "A dialogue between practitioners of alternative (traditional) medicine and modern (Western) medicine in Norway", in: *Social Science and Medicine*, 32(5): 549-552.

    1991b   *Den Andre Medisinen* (The Other Medicine), The University Press: Oslo.

Eisenberg, L.
    1977   "Disease and illness: distinctions between professional and popular ideas of sickness", in: *Cult. Med. Psychiat.*, 1: 9-23.

Fulder, S.
    1987   "Complementary medicine", in: *The Courier* (UNESCO), 40: 16-19.

Goffman, E.
    1959   *The Presentation of Self in Everyday Life*, Doubleday & Company: Garden City, New York.

Helman, C.
    1984   *Culture, Health and Illness. An Introduction for Health Professionals*, Wright: Bristol.

Illich, I. J.
    1974   *Energy and Equity*, Harper and Row: New York.

Ingstad, Benedicte
    1989   "Healer, Witch, Prophet or Modern Health-Worker? The Changing Role of Ngaka ya Setswana", in: A. J. Widing and A. Vesterlund (eds.), *Culture, Experience and Pluralism. Uppsala Studies in Cultural Anthropology*, Almqvist and Wiksell: Stockholm.

Karoliussen, M.
    1988   "Norsk Helsevesen – legeutdanning og verdier" (Norwegian Health Authority – education of doctors and values), in: *Tidsskrift Norske Lægeforening*, 108: 2747-2749.

Kleinman, A., Eisenberg, L. and Good, B.
    1978   "Culture, illness and care", in: *Ann. Intern. Med.* 88: 251-258.

Kleinman, A.
1980 "Patients and Healers in the Context of Culture", in: *An Exploration of the Borderland Between Anthropology, Medicine and Psychiatry*, University of California Press: Berkeley, CA.

Mahler, H.
1977 "The staff of Aesculapius", in: *World Health*, 3. Nov.

Malterud, K.
1987 "Illness and disease in female patients", in: *Scand. J. Prim. Health Care.*, 5: 205-209, 211-216.

Mills, T. M.
1967 *The Sociology of Small Groups*, Prentice Hall: New Jersey.

Sachs, L.
1983 "Evil eye or bacteria: turkish migrant women and swedish health care", in: *Studies in Social Anthropology*: Stockholm.

Sharma, U. M.
1990 Alternative Healing in a Midlands Locality. Report submitted to the Nuffield Foundation. April.

Alternative Therapy and Rationality

by Aase Krogh Mortensen

In this article I am going to make it my point that alternative therapy is rational, but that it is rational in another way than biomedicine. I am going to argue that the difference between alternative therapy and biomedicine can be considered a difference between two rationalities.

To talk about rationality in the plural would be considered something close to blasphemy only a few decades ago. The dominant opinion within science has been that there is only one rationality – and what does not conform to the standards of that rationality is by definition irrational.

What we consider to be irrational is very closely related to what we consider to be primitive, indicating that our frame of interpretation is deeply rooted in evolutionism.

The Construction of the Irrational

Within an evolutionary framework the scientist constructs a hierarchy between different cultures, with Western culture as the representative of culture in its highest and most civilized form. Other cultures are looked upon as expressions of Western culture in the past (Fabian 1983). For the evolutionist there are no real differences. There are only different stages of the same thing. Research on other cultures becomes research on the evolution of civilization as such.

A very dominant feature in "primitive" culture is found to be the inhabitants' inclination to magic. In fact, it is the flourishing of magic that is the paramount reason why these other cultures are called primitive (see Tylor 1903, Frazer 1911). Magic is seen as a rudimentary science. It is seen as primitive man's abortive attempt to create science – he tries to be rational, but he fails. It is within such a framework that the idea that all cultural expressions can be measured by the same standards of rationality has been conceived.

Even though the evolutionarily rooted approach to rationality still has its supporters, there seems to become more and more room for a broader conception of rationality. Within anthropology the evolutionary view lost most of its ground several decades ago, and the same seems to have happened in other academic disciplines. This change has a close connection with a general "crisis" in the conception of science. Some even speak of a paradigm shift. At least other conceptions of reality than the ones that belong to the positivistic paradigm, have become more visible within science. The idea that what does not conform to the standards of the positivistic paradigm is irrational and ripe for rejection is being challenged.

Today, it is becoming harder and harder to accept that large parts of what people do is being defined as irrational. And it is becoming more and more obvious that what we define as irrational is defined as such because it escapes the concepts of the hitherto dominant scientific paradigm. The fact that anthropologists talk about "otherness" instead of about irrationality is, as I see it, an expression of serious attempts to understand the kind of reality that escapes positivistic science. It is an attempt to understand it as something with a logic of its own.

The anthropological interest in "otherness" is primarily an interest in understanding how people live in other cultures. Even though anthropology has always been comparative, and the comparison with our own culture has always been – if not explicitly then implicitly – present, it is only recently it has become accepted to make Western culture the central concern of research.

It has become clear that "otherness" belongs to "us" as well (see for example Favret-Saada 1977, Luhrmann 1989, McGuire 1994), and if we compare this finding to the findings of anthropologists who have concentrated their academic interest on cultures not familiar with Western science, we see that at a very general level the difference between "us" and "them" is not radical. These writers have demonstrated that so-called primitive people are not totally swallowed up by magic. They actually do engage themselves in activities on the same logical ground as science (see Malinowski 1948, Evans-Pritchard 1976).

The universal simultaneity of magic and science cannot be explained within an evolutionary framework. Even though it might be suggested that the fact that so-called primitive people are able to act rationally (in a scientific sense) indicates that they are becoming aware of the flaws of magic – that it is a sign of development – the evolutionary framework simply leaves us mystified as to why magic should persist in our scientific Western culture, if it really just is a primitive version of science. A framework that can embrace magic and science as two different kinds of rationality, has a much better hold on the reported simultaneity.

Alternative Therapy and Biomedicine: Two Different Rationalities

One of the domains within Western culture where magic is flourishing is within the domain of alternative therapy. And as biomedicine relates to a positivistic (natural scientific) paradigm the contrast between the two domains is clear. But before I engage myself with a description of the relationship between alternative therapy and biomedicine as a relationship between two different rationalities, I find it necessary to point out, that it is only within a certain context that it makes sense to talk about the relationship between alternative therapy and biomedicine and the two rationalities in this either/or way.

It is when we focus on the self-defined differences between the two medical domains that are constructed in counterdistinction to each other, that it makes sense to talk about the relationship between the two domains as a relationship between the two rationalities. Alternative therapy is constructed as a critique of biomedicine (see McKee 1988). The fact that it is possible to talk about the richly faceted alternative therapies under one heading, is due to their shared reaction against biomedicine. Even though it would not be quite right to talk about biomedicine as constructed in counterdistinction to alternative therapy, as biomedicine existed prior to alternative therapy, it is nevertheless constructed in counterdistinction to magical medicine, that has always existed simultaneously with scientific medicine (see Hastrup 1989, Kleinman 1984).

The truths about the "self" and the "other" that are constructed in this process are not exact representations of reality. We could, in accordance with the American anthropologist James Boon (1982: 3-26), say that in the process of creating a cultural identity, the differences between the "self" and the "other" are exaggerated. The "other" becomes what the "self" is not and vice versa. The distinction between the two domains as a distinction between the two rationalities is constructed in this process.

It is thus my point that even though these exaggerated differences cannot be viewed as exact representations of reality, they can nevertheless be viewed as very active parts of reality. In other words, the self-defined differences are not only affected by reality. They also affect reality.

The biomedical doctor defines him- or herself in relation to a scientific rationality which leads his or her attention in a particular direction in the encounter with the patient. The positivistic paradigm orients the doctor towards analysis. Characteristic of this approach is a focus on dividing the world into parts considered to be autonomous entities. This framework leads the doctor to seek out the sick part or parts of the patient, and therapy then becomes an attack on the concrete manifestations of the patient's illness.

The alternative therapist defines him- or herself in relation to a magical rationality which leads him or her in quite another direction than the biomedical doctor. It leads him or her towards synthesis, where the focus is on the creation of relations and meaning in the world.

In such a world view the parts are nothing in themselves. They do not have fixed identities. Their identities change when the situation changes. You could say that the focus on relations and wholeness provides the parts with flexibility, so that their identity is under constant transformation.

This focus on wholeness leads the alternative therapist to go the opposite way of the biomedical doctor in seeking out the causes of illness. The concrete localized manifestations of the patient's illness are very often defined as symptoms of some deeper imbalance in the patient or in the relationship between the patient and the environment, or whatever makes sense to that particular therapist and patient, and in that particular therapeutic situation. This means that the same symptoms can be defined as having different causes in different patients.

The point is that the alternative therapist is concerned with linking together. The alternative therapist is concerned with helping the ill person create order in the chaotic situation that he or she experiences. The alternative therapist often sees him- or herself as a kind of catalyst, whose job it is to initiate a healing process in the patient and in his or her situation as a whole.

Even though we should not forget that all therapists (or for that matter all magicians and scientists) in some way or another and in different degrees relate to both rationalities, the fact that the biomedical doctor has his attention focused on analysis and the fact that the alternative therapist has his attention focused on synthesis creates a complementarity between the two medical domains. By consulting both alternative therapists and biomedical doctors the patient can act upon different aspects of the illness.

The magical approach to illness is just as valuable as the scientific. It is just different. An acknowledgement of this difference and of the complementarity between the two approaches must lead us to abandon the idea that the analytic approach is a "better" version and therefore qualified to measure the synthesizing approach. This would be an important step towards the construction of a health care system, where the synthesizing approach is not marginalized – a health care system where it enjoys official acceptance alongside the analytic approach.

References

Boon, J. A.
    1982   *Other Tribes, Other Scribes. Symbolic Anthropology in the Comparative Study of Cultures, Histories, Religions, and Texts*, Cambridge.

Evans-Pritchard, E. E.
    1976   *Witchcraft, Oracles and Magic among the Azande*, Clarendon Press: Oxford.

Fabian, J.
1983   *Time and the Other: How Anthropology Makes its Object,* Columbia University Press: New York.

Favret-Saada, J.
1977   *Les Mots, la Mort, les Sorts,* Gallimard.

Frazer, J. G.
1911   *The Golden Bough. The Magic Art and the Evolution of Kings,* Macmillan and Co.: London.

Hastrup, K.
1989   "Magi og videnskab", in: *Månedsskrift for Praktisk Lægegerning,* 67(10).

Kleinman, A.
1984   "Indigenous Systems of Healing: Questions for Professional, Popular, and Folk Care", in: J. Warren Salmon (ed.): *Alternative Medicine. Popular and Policy Perspectives,* Tavistock Publications: London.

Luhrmann, T. M.
1989   *Persuasion of the Witch's Craft. Ritual, Magic and Witchcraft in Present-day England,* Basil Blackwell: Oxford.

Malinowski, B.
1948   *Magic, Science & Religion and Other Essays,* The Free Press: London.

McGuire, M. B.
1994   *Ritual Healing in Suburban America,* Rutgers University Press: New Brunswick, New Jersey.

McKee, J.
1988   "Holistic health and the critique of Western medicine", in: *Soc. Sci. Med.,* 26(8).

Tylor, E. B.
1903   *Primitive Culture. Researches into the Development of Mythology, Philosophy, Religion, Language, Art, and Custom,* John Murray: London.

Communicating the Individual Body and the Body Politic

The discourse on disease prevention and health promotion in alternative therapies

by Espen Braathen

This paper is based on a small-scale study comprising extensive, semi-structured interviews with twenty-five practitioners of homoeopathy working in the two largest cities of Norway, Oslo and Bergen. The aim of the study is to examine the perceptions and constructions of disease prevention and health promotion in alternative therapies, particularly within homoeopathy.

The paper starts by introducing some central themes in the homoeopathic discourse on disease prevention and health promotion, paying particular attention to the construction of disease and the bodily expressions of symptoms. Health promotion is then discussed and defined within a comparative framework relating the homoeopathic ideas of health promotion to the conception of the phenomenon within the health promotion movement. The second part of the paper is concerned with the relationship between the body and the body politic[1] and asks whether health promotion in homoeopathy is a new form of panoptic vision or rather a strategy for empowering the patient.

My point of departure feeds on the conviction that the current discourse in alternative therapies is intrinsically woven into a modernist version of the cultural dialogue between science and religion, knowledge and faith, scepticism and energistic or spiritual principles for constructing the world and the body. This discourse is, thus, part of an ongoing cultural struggle for defining the dominant forms and meanings of science and medicine.

---

1 The body politic refers to the third level of Scheper-Hughes and Lock's (1987) conceptualization of the three bodies; the individual body, the social body and the body politic respectively. The last of which concerns the issues of power and control in the relationships between individual and social bodies. According to Scheper-Hughes and Lock "*an anthropology of relations between the body and the body politic inevitably leads to a consideration of the regulation and control not only of individuals but of populations...*" (Scheper-Hughes and Lock 1987: 27).

Carol MacCormac, writing on the holistic health movement, contends that *"people in increasing numbers appear to be viewing themselves and all being within a framework of wholeness and implicate order. This is a world view in direct contrast to that of allopathic medicine which is based on a diagnostic process which splits people down to a diseased organ, and uses drugs which induce an opposite condition as part of the cure – to correct the malfunctioning part"* (MacCormac 1991: 265).

The holistic health movement might be read as an embodied contestation of the ways in which people have come to see reality through a scientific lens and, hence, a quest for living in a culture, to quote MacCormac again, *"which is simultaneously enriched by magic, religion and science, harmonised within a unified world view"* (MacCormac 1991: 268).

The biological reductionism of biomedicine which tends to reduce the whole person to its physical body has become increasingly difficult to accept wholeheartedly for most people (Benoist and Cathebras 1993). People tend to accept biological knowledge per se but they do not accept a purely biological conception of their own bodies. They conceive that there must be an immaterial part of the human body. This part, however, is not necessarily a supernatural one, but might be as in the homoeopathic discourse integral to nature.

Homoeopathy

The homoeopathic practitioners' narratives of disease prevention and health promotion are closely related to a discourse of nature, wholeness and principles of the energistic body. All of which is spun around Hahnemann's axiom that *"all diseases are, in fact, diseases of the whole organism."* One homoeopath suggested to me that *"the use of homoeopathic remedies is also part of the process of restoring the balance of the remedy and, as such, homoeopathy is actually involved in healing the whole world."* Another homoeopath insisted that the remedies prescribed worked, according to not yet discovered natural laws, saying that *"it is important to allow nature itself to put things straight"*. Nature is, in this context, to be understood as a physical reality, but one which is 'illuminated' by an omnipresent energy. The discourse on nature and natural ways of curing becomes important in homoeopathy as nature and the individual body are seen as a whole; part and parcel of the same energistic organism.

Symptoms are in the homoeopathic discourse the natural primal language of the body through which the disease 'talks' to the homoeopath. Because the disease, according to homoeopathic theory, is unknowable, its causes are neither known to man by the eye or by the microscope. Hence, the body's symptomatology is the only way in which to express and respond to an underlying disturbance. *"Its response"*, as Grossinger notes, *"is actually a system-wide recognition of the existence of disease within itself and a synchronous attempt to allow the disease . . . to express and vent itself with the least damage to the vital organs"* (Grossinger 1980: 170).

The natural ways of curing, based upon Hahnemann's Law of Similars and Hering's Law,[2] also guide the homoeopathic discourse on disease prevention and health promotion. Before embarking on this issue it is necessary to briefly outline what is to be understood by these concepts.

Health Promotion and Homoeopathy

According to the tenets of the new public health movement[3] it is the effect of the total environment on health which is of concern, for as much as socio-ecological and politico-economic issues seem to gain the upper hand over individualised health enhancing strategies. Don Nutbeam, writing from his position within the new public health establishment, defines disease prevention as representing *"strategies designed either to reduce risk-factors for specific disease, or to enhance host factors that reduce susceptibility to disease"* (Nutbeam 1986: 115). Such strategies, focusing on groups at risk and diseases, have been met with substantial critique, however, not least from medical anthropologists (Farmer 1992, Schiller 1992, 1994, Singer 1994), for blaming the victim and isolating disease disposing factors from their wider socio-cultural environment.

Health promotion, on the other hand, starts out with a vision of health as a resource for everyday life and focuses on the whole population in the context of their daily activities. Thus, the World Health Organization defines health promo-

---

[2] Hering's Law refers to the influential work of Hahnemann's follower Constantine Hering who developed notions about the specific order of curative sequences in homoeopathy. According to Hering a cure proceeds from the top down and from the inside out. Furthermore, when a cure is in progress the symptoms disappear in the reverse order of their appearance.

[3] The new public health movement emerged in the 1970s and was a response to the twentieth century's general preoccupation with individual health. The new public health wants to regenerate the original public health movement of the nineteenth century and its focus on interventions at environmental infrastructures affecting health (Bunton and Macdonald 1992). Deborah Lupton contends that the history of *"the 'new' public health is typically represented as a reaction against both the individualistic and victim blaming approach of health education and the curative model of biomedicine. It is heralded as a return to the concern with environmental factors that first generated the public health movement of the nineteenth century. . . . Health promotion is a central plank of the 'new' public health"* (Lupton 1995: 50).

tion as *"the process of enabling people to increase control over, and to improve, their health"* (WHO 1986). In order to carry out such an ambitious task health promotion actions work:

- to build healthy public policies;
- to create supportive environments;
- to strengthen community action;
- to develop personal skills; and
- to reorient health services.

Strategies which together stress the collective efforts to attain, maintain and reproduce health. Health promotion and disease prevention are frequently used synonymously but have to be seen as two separate, though complementary, strategies in the fight for public health (Chapman and Lupton 1994). This fight is, as Foucault (1984) has convincingly argued, fed by the modern state's preoccupation with controlling and shaping bodies.

Moving on to the homoeopathic discourse on these issues, it should become clear from the discussion which follows, that this professional group of therapists shares common ground with the health promotion movement. The homoeopathic view of disease prevention and health promotion is, as would be expected, solidly rooted in the therapeutic encounter and is, as such, basically an individualised strategy in which the individual body becomes the locus nexus for enhancing health.

As a leading homoeopath related to me: *"The homoeopathic interview is extremely important, and a solution to most problems is to be found here ... If the person had a better understanding of himself or herself this would radically improve the public health."* Societal, or structural, disease-disposing and health-enabling factors, and their importance, are not misconceived or denied by the homoeopaths, but as one homoeopath said to me: *"It is really nothing we can do at this level of causation."* There is a widespread belief in the homoeopathic discourse, however, that these factors will be reflected in the picture of symptoms which is always the endpoint of any therapeutic encounter, and which the therapist and patient are obliged to work on in order to disclose.

It would be true to say that the homoeopaths have a clear, but rarely explicit, understanding and formulation of the structural constraints set by the body politic in matters concerning health. The homoeopathic line of argument emphasises that the potencised remedy prescribed to the patient has the potential to effect processes of change which means that when the patient starts to get better he or she might go through an ontological transformation which has the power to alter the patient's relationship to both his or her individual body, and the social body. As one homoeopath told me: *"If the remedy hits the right strings it might revolutionise the patient's life."*

Cure and health promotion go hand in hand and are, indeed, inseparable. Curative actions always have a preventive aim, namely to strengthen the patient's vital force to such an extent that the organism can rid itself of the problems that restrict the person. One homoeopath puts it like this: *"Right treatment of a patient will always have a preventive effect. It strengthens the defence system in such a way as to enable the person to become less susceptible to disease."*

There is, however, another important and closely related thread running through the homoeopathic discourse which attests to the strong belief in raising the consciousness of the patient in matters of health and illness, and in particular to encourage the patient to take responsibility for his or her own health. One homoeopath suggested that *"homoeopathy is a relatively cheap and simple form of cure but it does, indeed, demand active participation and commitment from the patient."* The issue of personal responsibility for health will be dealt with, but first I want to go back to what constitutes the common ground of homoeopathy and health promotion.

Both homoeopathy and health promotion share a deep scepticism towards the biomedical model which is basically focused on disease and grounded in, what Gordon (1988) calls, some "tenacious assumptions" concerning naturalism, individualism and reductionism which reproduce the dualistic thought system so deeply embedded in Western culture.

The focus on health, on the other hand, which characterises the approaches of homoeopathy and health promotion celebrates health as a positive value stressing its potential for achieving freedom and well-being.

Furthermore, both of the latter disapprove of the harmful effects of medicine, and in particular the iatrogenic disturbances caused by overmedication. Empowerment or the process of enabling people to achieve their fullest health potential is another important issue in both discourses.

Finally, emphasis is put on a holistic approach which is seen as essential for transcending the traditional biomedical model of disease and for realising health. However, the issue of holism is also the line which divides the two camps. Wholeness in the homoeopathic discourse is limited to the individual body, although this body is perceived as a total energy complex comprising a mental-spiritual plane, an emotional-psychic plane, and a physical plane which all attach to the all-embracing organism of nature (Vithoulkas 1991).

Health promotion, on the other hand, adheres to the WHO's construction of wholeness as incorporating the physical, mental and social, thus paying attention to both the individual and the social body. There is, however, an emergent tendency in the health promotion discourse to account for the importance of the body politic. A focus which seems totally lacking in the homoeopathic discourse.

Health Promotion in Homoeopathy: Panoptic Vision?

One of the least explained let alone researched topics in the anthropology of alternative medicine is the relation between the body and the body politic which inevitably leads to questions of power and control. Ursula Sharma, for instance, discussing the therapeutic encounter and the differences between what happens in the consulting room of the GP and the homoeopath respectively, states that *"to the extent that the complementary practitioner usually operates quite independently of the state's interest in the bodies and health of its citizens there is always the potential for a very radical difference. Most complementary practice does not (at present) participate in the panoptical surveillance of citizens envisaged by Foucault"* (Sharma 1994: 102).

I would suggest that such a reading of Foucault is incomplete as his conception of disciplinary power, worked into subtle technologies of the self, clearly points in the direction of harnessing bodies that are linked together in invisible relational networks and, as such, are unaware of its geometrical site of power and control.

Similarly, Norbert Elias (1939/1994) has suggested that power and power relations are interdependent ties intrinsic to the civilizing process and the development of a body politic. It is interesting, with these perspectives in mind, to make a brief excursion into the highly relevant question of medicalisation, understood as the process of labelling normal bodily functions and social issues as problems requiring medical solutions.

Nancy Scheper-Hughes and Margaret Lock writing on this topic emphasize *"the usefulness to the body politic of filtering more and more human unrest, dissatisfaction, longing, and protest into the idiom of sickness, which can be safely managed by doctor-agents"* (Scheper-Hughes and Lock 1987: 27). The stability of the body politic rests precisely on its ability to produce docile, though flexible bodies, as Martin (1994) adds, conforming to the needs of the social and political order. Medicalisation is, thus, a powerful strategy by which culturally specific definitions and meanings of health and social well-being are passed on and reproduced.

Homoeopaths oppose what they see as the medicalisation of life and the hegemony of the doctor on the grounds that it deflects the person from understanding the wider mental-spiritual and emotional-psychic causes of health and robs the individual of the responsibility for his or her own health development.

Instead, they focus their gaze on health, promoting an option of gentleness (Douglas 1994) and personal responsibility. It would not be too farfetched to suggest that the homoeopathic discourse constructs a new kind of medicalisation through 'healthisation' of life as every aspect of the patient's life is of interest in establishing a complete symptom picture. This might be termed a new form of surveillance of life-worlds, where the homoeopath has become an important agent in putting into effect self-disciplining technologies.

Technologies of the self are gentle in a political sense by procuring valuable information about the patient, unavailable to national health statistics, but which strengthen the grip on private life-worlds and depoliticise the work on health. The homoeopath is, moreover, in the therapeutic encounter and the work on the patient's health, consciously or unconsciously, conveying powerful images of the current social and political order as participant in a collective fight for public health.

In order to contextualise the dominant discourse on health in homoeopathy I will briefly discuss the heightened awareness and commercialisation of health in consumer capitalism (Barsky 1988, Crawford 1984, Saltonstall 1993).

Ulrich Beck (1992) has developed the notion of the 'risk society' in which he points out the transformation that has taken place, due to modernisation processes, with regard to the problem of risk. A general lesson imparted by his study refers to the fact that as the natural causes of risks have been reduced the man-made risks have dramatically increased in modern society. Accordingly, the consumer has been increasingly more concerned with issues of risk and how to control or manage risks. Such a view is closely related to contemporary concerns with health issues, both from the perspective of the new public health and alternative therapies, as they all work on health in order to minimise the risk of diseases.

What distinguishes this gaze from the more traditional, biomedically based strategies of preventive medicine and public health is that bodies are now controlled under the new idioms of freedom and empowerment. Alternative therapies, as well as the new public health movement, also seem to invoke theories which are global, holistic, spiritual or ecological in nature, rather than the local, partial and physical classifications and theories of preventive medicine and public health. Furthermore, as consumption of commodities has become central to how people define themselves, the body and the work on health have come to be regarded as consumer commodities competing to maximise their market value.

Robert Crawford's study (1984), and Saltonstall's study (1993) almost a decade later, have examined the lay notions of health in the North American population. Both studies underline the importance of self-control, discipline and deliberate, intentional actions in order to achieve health and improve one's bodily capital (Wacquant 1995). Crawford's study reinforces a critique launched in one of his earlier studies of the new health consciousness and health movements (1980), in which he showed how the construction of health in the holistic health, self-care and self-help movements has been primarily concerned with a discourse on the individual body.

This discourse which he terms 'healthism', describing the belief or cultural value that health is the prime object of living, privatises the struggle for societal well-being and thus reproduces, like the biomedical system, hegemonic values stressing individual responsibility for matters concerning health and disease.

... or Empowering Strategies?

In contrast to the disembodied discourse of preventive medicine and public health on health promotion, homoeopathy has located its discourse in the lives of patients evolving an embodied form of extraction of patient data. As suggested this constitutes a new kind of surveillance in which spiritual, psychological and emotional factors become increasingly important in a regime of discipline and regulation rather than the physical and social issues characterising the medico-social survey.

However, this type of power/knowledge production is an ambiguous one. The nature of its dialectic, stressing the notion of personal responsibility for health, is at the same time the source of empowering strategies. Empowerment, defined as *"the notion of people having to take action to control and enhance their own lives, and the process of enabling them to do so"* (Grace 1991: 330), has become the dominant aim and symbol of health promoting strategies. What the homoeopaths are doing both in the therapeutic encounter and by prescribing remedies is in fact perceived as empowering actions. As one homoeopath puts it: *"We (the homoeopaths) must help the patient to a fuller and more adequate life"*, or in the words of another: *"Homoeopathy contributes to a harmonious development of the person in his or her own surroundings."*

The 'optical' image Sharma (1994) is referring to of the homoeopath seeing himself or herself as a mirror reflecting back an image of the patient's life, represents a metaphor of the Law of Similars which I often came across in my interviews. The importance of invoking reactions in the patient's body during the therapeutic encounter, that are similar to his or her symptoms, is rendered vital, in fuelling the healing process. The therapist thus occupies an essential role in enabling the patient to take control of and enhance his or her own life and health.

Conclusion

Throughout the paper it has been an explicit aim to examine how power and control necessarily have to be important issues in the discourse on health promotion in homoeopathy. The dialectic of this discourse clearly shows how the production of power/knowledge in homoeopathy balances between the surveillance and regulation of citizens, and promoting empowering strategies for enhancing health.

The individualised strategy of empowerment in homoeopathy pays limited attention to the social and, indeed, politico-economic determinants necessary for facilitating changes in the factors which restrict the person. The homoeopathic strategies of empowering the patient are firmly rooted in the therapeutic encounter and the prescription of remedies. Both are fundamental to the homoeopathic understanding of the potentials as well as limitations of homoeopathic interventions. The homoeopathic contribution to improving the public health passes basically through individualised actions in which each person's individual symptom picture is the key to cure and attaining health.

In conclusion, it is worth noticing the way in which the medical gaze of homoeopathy is enacted. As the physical examination of the patient plays only a very limited role in the homoeopathic therapeutic encounter the making of the body takes a somewhat different direction from that described by Foucault (1976). According to Foucault the medical body was made into a static object which could be explored and examined according to the spatialisation of its surface dimensions, its anatomy and its social space. The homoeopathic discourse constructs an energistic body; a living, flexible organism which adopts and responds to its environment. Its responses can be read through the body's production of symptoms by invoking the individual body's self-healing energies by prescribing potencised homoeopathic remedies.

References

Beck, Ulrich
1992   *Risk Society. Towards a New Modernity*, Sage: London.

Barsky, A.J.
1988   "The paradox of health", in: *The New England Journal of Medicine*, 318 (7): 414-418.

Benoist, Jean and Pascal Cathebras
1993   "The body: from an immateriality to another", in: *Social Science and Medicine*, 36 (7): 857-865.

Bunton, Robin and Gordon Macdonald
1992 "Health Promotion: Discipline or Disciplines?", in: R. Bunton and G. Macdonald (eds.): *Health Promotion: Disciplines and Diversity*, Routledge: London.

Chapman, Simon and Deborah Lupton
1994 *The Fight for Public Health. Principles and Practice of Media Advocacy*, BMJ Publishing Group: London.

Crawford, Robert
1980 "Healthism and the medicalisation of everyday life", in: *International Journal of Health Services*, 10(3): 365-388.
1984 "A Cultural Account of 'Health': Control, Release, and the Social Body", in: J. B. McKinlay (ed.): *Issues in the Political Economy of Health Care*, pp. 61-103, Tavistock: London.

Douglas, Mary
1994 The construction of the physician: a cultural approach to medical fashion, in: S. Budd and U. Sharma (eds.): *The Healing Bond. The Patient-Practitioner Relationship and Therapeutic Responsibility*, pp. 23-41, Routledge: London.

Elias, Norbert
1994 *The Civilizing Process*, Blackwell: Oxford (1939).

Farmer, Paul
1992 *AIDS and Accusation. Haiti and the Geography of Blame*, The University of California Press: Berkeley.

Foucault, Michel
1976 *The Birth of the Clinic: An Archaeology of Medical Perception*, Tavistock: London.
1984 "The Politics of Health in the Eighteenth Century", in: P. Rabinow (ed.): *The Foucault Reader*, Penguin: London.

Gordon, Deborah
1988 "Tenacious Assumptions in Western Medicine", in: M. Lock and D. Gordon (eds.): *Biomedicine Examined*, Kluwer: Dordrecht.

Grace, Victoria M.
1991 "The marketing of empowerment and the construction of the health consumer: a critique of health promotion", in: *International Journal of Health Services*, 21(2): 329-343.

Grossinger, Richard
1980 *Planet Medicine. From Stone Age Shamanism to Post-Industrial Healing*, Shambhale: London.

Lupton, Deborah
1995 *The Imperative of Health. Public Health and the Regulated Body*, Sage: London.

MacCormac, Carol P.
1991 "Holistic health and a changing western world view", in: *Curare*, 7: 259-273.

Martin, Emily
1994 *Flexible Bodies. Tracking Immunity in American Culture from the Days of Polio to the Age of AIDS*, Beacon Press: Boston.

Nutbeam, Don
1986   "Health promotion glossary", in: *Health Promotion*, 1(1): 113-127.

Saltonstall, R.
1993   "Healthy bodies, social bodies: men's and women's concepts and practices of health in everyday life", in: *Social Science and Medicine*, 36(1): 7-14.

Scheper-Hughes, Nancy and Margaret M. Lock
1987   "The mindful body: a prolegomenon to future work in medical anthropology", in: *Medical Anthropology Quarterly*, 1(1): 6-41.

Schiller, Nina G.
1992   "What's wrong with this picture? The hegemonic construction of culture in AIDS research in the United States", in: *Medical Anthropology Quarterly*, 6(3): 237-245.
1994   "Risky business: the cultural construction of AIDS risk groups", in: *Social Science and Medicine*, 38(10): 1337-1346.

Singer, Merrill
1994   "AIDS and the health crisis of the U.S. urban poor: the perspective of critical medical anthropology", *Social Science and Medicine*, 39(7): 931-948.

Vithoulkas, George
1991   *A New Model of Health and Disease*, North Atlantic Books: Berkeley.

Wacquant, Loic J.D.
1995   "Pugs at work: bodily capital and bodily labour among professional boxers", in: *Body and Society*, 1(1): 65-93.

World Health Organization
1986   *The Ottawa Charter for Health Promotion*, Ottawa/Copenhagen: WHO.

In the Twilight Zone

A personal report from a medical doctor betwixt and between

by Bent Eikard

The title means that I am in the process – that I am still working at the relationship between orthodox medicine and alternative medicine:

- should they be bridged? – integrated? (which into which?)
- should they complement each other? – or is that impossible?
- should the two fields of treatment just learn to accept each other without necessarily understanding each other and live peacefully together (which has been possible for some religions in some cultures for some time through the history of mankind)?
- should the one extinguish the other? – and who should it then be that "survived"?
- should it all become "official" – but who should decide the rules for that?
- and what should be the economic consequences? – and wouldn't there always be something "alternative"?
- or is it all hopeless because there are so many emotions involved in these questions and both orthodox and alternative medicine are so closed that we can hardly speak of communication?

Medical doctors and alternative therapists seldom meet each other personally. They hear and read about each other and fight each other in organizations, court rooms and the media.

As an anesthesiologist and pain therapist in private practice I know how difficult and painful life can be – and how extremely difficult it can be to help fellow human beings. Through my clinical experience, I have learned that everything in this universe is connected somehow. And if one would do good work with patients in pain, one should be ready to look at the patients' situation and treatment not only biologically – but also psychologically, politically, socio-culturally, intellectually, and from the viewpoint of different belief systems and different premature cognitive commitments, religions, feelings, spiritual and artistic expressions.

One thing that helped me enormously to survive all the sickness, the suffering, the pain, the fear of death, with which I have been presented through the years, is to adopt a humorous distance in an attempt not to be cynical nor to burn out. Of course this is a balance too: I am not talking about being ironic or sarcastic – but about warm humour combined with compassion and love. It is a difficult art and sometimes I make mistakes.

With humor in the baggage it is also easier to avoid fanaticism. I see a fanatic as an idealist without humor – or an idealist as a fanatic with humor! And I would rather see myself as an idealist than a fanatic. I try to learn not to take things too seriously and try to make a game out of most of what I am doing. Sometimes I do not succeed – which gives me quite a lot of pain! And of course I want to be taken seriously myself – even when I am joking! A joke can be a very serious matter.

Now and then, I am a little frightened of what could be called "neo-fascism". A phenomenon I observe in certain circles interested in therapy and health – both within orthodox medicine and alternative medicine. More or less transparent manipulations are used to get people to live certain lifestyles, either through official campaigns or during private consultations.

"Everyone is his own responsibility – choose what you want to be" is one of my favorite sayings. Hearing this, people might ask: What can we then do for each other?

We can give some help and try to get our fellow human beings to help themselves the rest of the way, through taking the responsibility for their own lives by stimulating their own inner life forces. For the good doctor or alternative therapist it is the therapeutic decision when the help should stop and the self-help begin. Sometimes we ask too much of patients (and children and partners and colleagues etc.) and they may break down. And sometimes we claim too little and they might get spoiled. As Ovid put it: *"Pars sanitatis velle sanari"* (it is part of the healing that you want to be healed). I usually put it this way: Only you can do it (but maybe it is not always possible for you to do it alone). It is my experience that if people feel good they mostly have themselves to blame!

Sickness

When I went to medical school we were almost only trained in dealing with sickness. We never heard of health in any other sense than not being sick meant being healthy! And so it continued through my first 10 years of clinical experience. I was so indoctrinated at the university that I more focused on medical *science*, dealing with sickness and treatment, than medical *art*, dealing with health and empathy. Diagnosis of sickness was interesting – health was just normal and a little boring. Gradually, I discovered that the health care system in itself might somehow be sick: It called itself *health* care but dealt nearly only with *sickness!*

97% of the budget of the Danish health care system is spent on treating sickness – and only 3% on prophylactic work. But who would fly with an airline using 97% of its turnover on repairing aeroplanes that had fallen down, instead of using 97% trying to avoid crashes?

Of course a little is done prophylactically, but it goes very slowly. That's the reason why some have renamed the WHO-project "Health for all at year 2000" to: "Health for all in 2000 years"! The general attitude seems to be that the doctors and the health care system are waiting for sickness instead of actively trying to avoid it.

In ancient China, it seemed to be different (for those who could afford to have a doctor at all!). In an old Chinese textbook, "The Yellow Emperor's Nei Ching" (a classic of internal medicine from the 2nd century BC), we can read: *"The wise doctor does not wait until people get sick. He guides them when they are in good health by giving them good advice. In this way he gets them to flourish continuously."* The word *"flourish"* never occurred in my medical textbooks at the university!

Health

After all my years with sicknesses I got sick of sickness and started to look at and work with healthy people to try to get them to stay healthy. Nobody plans to get sick. Everybody wants to be healthy and rich – not sick and poor! So what is happening when we get sick anyway? I often see reasons like ignorance of the consequences of what we are doing to our lives, lack of strength or indolence or laziness – or pure self-destruction. Somebody said that from a certain point of view this hidden form of slow suicide seems to be the most common cause of premature death in Denmark.

Practically everybody in a country like Denmark knows how to eat in a healthy way, that exercise is essential, as is getting enough sleep etc. etc. We know the official paths to a healthy life – but only a few follow them thoroughly. Why? I think that one important reason is that such claims are often very boring and presented in a fanatic and self-righteous way!

There is this saying: *It's not necessarily fun to live in a healthy way – but it's always healthy to live in a fun way!* Most people want a good life rather than a healthy one as defined by experts and authorities. The thing is to unite these two ways of living into one. And everyone is responsible for doing that in his own way.

The attitude of the old Eastern medical universe was that trying to treat disease was like forging weapons after the war had started. In ancient China colleagues ideally estimated each other according to the following criteria: The good doctors' clients did not get sick. The mediocre doctors' clients could get sick, but they could then cure them. The bad doctors' clients got sick – and they could not cure them.

The concept we see here is the good doctor as a custodian of health. The above mentioned definition of the bad doctor seems to describe the situation of many doctors and alternative therapists today. As one of my friends told me a while ago: *"I do not think my doctor is especially good – all his clients are in bad health!"*

The old Eastern ideal is the opposite of the description Voltaire gave of the state of the art for doctors and medical science some 250 years ago: *"Doctors are people who give medicine they do not know much about for diseases they know less about to fellow beings they know nothing about"*. Or: *"Medical science or medical art is the science or the art of keeping people distracted with different doings of no use until nature has either cured them or killed them."*

This description is still pertinent to a lot of situations within orthodox as well as alternative medicine.

Orthodox Medicine

The dominant, scientifically based medical model is in many ways incomplete. But of course it also has gained a lot of valuable victories in this century for which it should be credited – especially in situations of acute disease and surgery.

But:
- about 1/3 of people in contact with the official health care systems in Western societies today also get so-called iatrogenic diseases (diseases made by doctors through diagnostic and therapeutic procedures) that complicate their disease situation to some degree – sometimes seriously.

- many people die of resistant infections caught in hospitals – a situation which seems to be getting worse because of an uncritical use of antibiotics.

- addiction to legally prescribed medical drugs has gone up by 300% in the last few years, while addiction to illegal street drugs has only increased 30%.

A Harvard sociologist has pointed out that the amount of pain and agony caused by the technical medical treatment in the US nearly reached the level of suffering caused by traffic accidents, work place accidents – and even war related activity!

All these drawbacks and side effects together make modern medicine one of the fastest growing epidemics, it has been said.

Alternative Medicine

When I started my travels towards new medical horizons – moving my body around the world and concepts around in my head – I do not really know what expectations I had. I was just a searching soul looking for alternatives, forced, among other things, by frustrations with my pain work, which in mainstream medicine has a rather low status as it is nearly impossible to measure physical pain in an objective way – not to mention the sorrow, anxiety and depression connected to it.

With no other real expectations than finding something new and reviving, I was disappointed to find so much of the same old stuff in the alternative area that I was tired of in the orthodox medical world:

- I saw a lot of alternative therapists fighting and mistrusting each other even more than doctors do – and I was surprised to see how often they dressed like doctors and used different technical machinery and talked about "scientific proof".
- I saw a lot of alternative therapists from quite different areas who claimed to know the whole truth and be the (only) truly holistics – even if they did not in my opinion at all take everything into account or look at the whole picture.
- I saw a lot of therapists who saw things only from their own point of view, and in their intolerance to others even refused to look more closely at other "alternatives".
- I tried to work in integrated centres of orthodox and alternative medicine – but we did not succeed because we either would not listen to each other or did not understand each other.
- I found a lot of poor education, quackery and money making.
- I often found very authoritarian therapeutic behaviour, leaving the patient only two choices: Take it or leave it!
- I found a lack of interest in searching for new and better ways in many alternative therapies: because they were perfect as they were and were grounded on dogmas which could not be subject to scientifically based doubt and curiosity. Dogmas which I often saw as nearly religious.

But I also found the following advantages of alternative medicine. It:

- often has simple, non-technical diagnostic procedures.
- has reduced costs (of treatment and diagnosis).
- has little or no side effects.
- often allows more time for and interest in the patient in humanistic, non-bureaucratic and non-institutionalized settings and considers the patient an individual, a unique person.
- often focuses more on the patient's strength and health than on sickness.
- has cosmologies which are much different from the scientific one. They seem more "human", broad and warm to people as they include feelings and bring spirituality into therapy.
- has many therapists who speak the same language and are on the same (social) level with their patients – while academic, scientifically trained doctors often are talking a quite different language, are living in another world and have a quite different (scientific) world view which scientifically untrained people do not understand.

Communication between Orthodox Medicine and Alternative Medicine

Holistic medicine
In the theory of holism the whole organism and its systems are greater than the sum of their parts. Holistic medicine addresses not only the whole person, but also the person's environment and involves various healing and health-promoting practices. In the last decade the holistic health movement has witnessed an increase in popularity and acceptance, and the holistic philosophy has expanded into the field of medicine.

There are three basic aspects of the holistic approach to medicine: First, it emphasizes disease prevention by placing responsibility with the individual as self-healer – to use his own resources to promote health, prevent illness, and encourage healing. Holistic practitioners believe that patients should be active participants in their own health care since all individuals are believed to have the capacity – mental, emotional, social, spiritual, and physical – to heal themselves. Second, holistic medicine considers the patient an individual and a unique person, not a symptom-bearing organism. Finally, holistic practitioners attempt to make use of the many available diagnoses, treatments, and health methods, including both alternative and standard medical methods. Holistic health practitioners view the use of standard medical practices as only one of many ways in which to achieve well-being.

Holistic diagnosis may include standard laboratory tests or other diagnostic methods. The interrelated physical, mental, and spiritual capabilities in the whole person are major health determinants. A practitioner may, for example, watch the way patients stand, sit, and walk, as well as look for the physical expression of an emotional state. Health-care treatments are usually provided in the context of the patient's culture, family, and community.

Once an illness has been identified, it is viewed both as a misfortune and an opportunity for discovery. Holistic medicine emphasizes the idea that psychosocial stresses, such as unemployment, divorce, or death of a close relative or friend, may contribute to ill health.

In recent years, a variety of traditionally trained medical professionals have examined the ideals and documented benefits of holistic medicine. Some still criticize the fragmentation of the holistic medical movement and blame it for promoting medical quackery. Others, calling for physicians to appear as consolers and healers as well as technologically trained practitioners, embrace the humanistic approach offered by holistic medicine. The means by which a cure is produced is not nearly so important as the fact that the cure is produced!

Can it be done?
Is it, generally speaking, possible to bridge the "gap" between orthodox and alternative medicine? How can a gap between different cosmologies (or paradigms) be bridged? Does it mean a) to try to integrate them or let them supplement each other like in holistic medicine as described above? or b) does "bridging" mean to try to get these often totally different worlds to peacefully accept each other's existence (also officially) whether they understand each other or not – and let people make their own choices?

Considering the former, can different cosmologies be united, integrated or supplement each other without compromising – at least some of and maybe all of – their own essential nature and thereby their uniqueness and strength? Is it at all possible to make a "new cosmology" or "new paradigm" stronger and more comprehensive than the existing ones? – or is Kipling still pertinent as a metaphor in saying *"East is east and west is west . . . ?"*

Regarding the latter, if we – as a principle – had a situation of mutual acceptance, it could be the first step towards a more elaborated bridging based on a more extended understanding of each other's worlds. As the British Medical Journal put it in the heading of an article about these questions: *"Doctors and witchdoctors: Which doctors are which?"*

I personally find it obvious that we should try to harmonize the relationship between orthodox medicine and alternative medicine and learn from each other and complement each other's knowledge as far as possible. Orthodox medicine and alternative medicine should unite to identify the best part of the alternative therapists and establish some kind of authorization schedule with certain professional criteria to be fulfilled before authorization and official economic support.

The scientific situation

Many kinds of alternative medicine seem to me to be traditions based on dogmas close to religious belief systems and therefore not necessarily interested in scientific research as there is no need of revision. Alternative therapists often "know" (believe, hope) beforehand that their kind of treatment will work. So research is superfluous and sometimes even considered unethical. That which should be investigated is taken for granted. Religion – which is faith – excludes science – which is critical. Science is even self-critical. They are two different areas – which might learn to live together but cannot be integrated in one concept.

Alternative medicine lacks a comprehensive evaluation of its efficacy and socio-cultural impact. Therefore, alternative medicine in general is sparsely represented in research at universities. An additional characteristic of this field is that it is not fully covered in the usual scientific literature data banks and that it is difficult to obtain overviews on research progress.

Healing

Healing the sick – the practice of medicine – is one of the oldest professional callings. From ancient times persons with medical skills have tried to ease the distress of the ailing. But as Hippocrates put it: *The doctor treats – nature heals.*

Personally, I first and foremost want to mobilize the individual's self-healing capacity. I emphasize disease prevention by trying to inspire people to take responsibility and by making the individual patient a self-healer – to use his own resources to promote health, prevent illness, and encourage healing. A treatment should in principal work better through stimulation of the self-healing capacity of the organism than as a result of pharmacological intervention.

We know deep inside us how our lives ought to be lived – we know that without help from anybody. But we do not seek out peaceful surroundings much to listen to ourselves in Western societies. If we did, we would learn that life knows how to survive as a result of its development through millions and millions of years.

In a way one can say that *we* are billions of years old through the information stored in the DNA molecule in our cells. And the stuff we are made of is even older as we are made of stardust! We can say we are as old as the universe! So life has – or we have – some kind of experience we must say!

My point here is that as we (life) represent such an old knowledge we somehow must know within ourselves how to live and how to survive all the dangers we are surrounded by: Life must know how to survive somehow – even without doctors, therapists and all other kinds of specialists. We might not need experts or therapists as we could serve as our own best expert. We *know* because we are alive!

The placebo response
When I went to medical school we were taught that the phenomena of *the placebo response*[1] or *the nocebo response*[2] was something disturbing and without interest – something to be excluded. And the technique to do so was the controlled, randomized, double or triple blind clinical trial. But in fact the placebo or nocebo responses are highly interesting. *What is going on here?*

It has recently been discovered that we have, in our cells, specific receptors for all kinds of biochemicals. Medicine only works if we have specific receptors for it in our body. But if we have specific receptors for specific chemicals it must be because we ourselves can make the specific chemicals for those specific receptors. We do not have specific receptors because we have a contract with the medicinal industry to produce certain drugs for those receptors!

In other words: The placebo response – as we can see in varying percentages between 5-95% depending on which medicine or treatment (even operations) we want to examine – seems to indicate that we can make all kinds of "medicine" and have all kinds of rebuilding systems at our disposal in our body. We have an inner pharmacy, so to speak, combined with a "know how" or "understanding" about how to use it.

This inner knowledge of surviving – and not only surviving, but living a good and long life – was put into words and formulated in scriptures through a process of inner, meditative cognition by sages in the old Indian culture. They called it *Ayur Veda* – meaning "The science of life", a medical system still alive and widely accepted by WHO and a growing number of Western trained doctors.

---

1 Understood as manifestations of positive, expected or wanted effects without pharmacological or other physical influences.
2 Understood as manifestations of negative, feared or unwanted effects without pharmacological or other physical influences.

Our life potentialities
In our days Ayur Veda could also be called the knowledge or the science of the *survival potential of life* [3] – an essential part of which is the *healing potential*. Life wants to survive. It is the nature of life to expand and enjoy. If we combine this with the precondition that we have a *free will* (within certain more or less wide limits) we reach the conclusion: The more free will, the more *choices* and the more *responsibility*. This gives us basically the choice between whether we want to live or not.

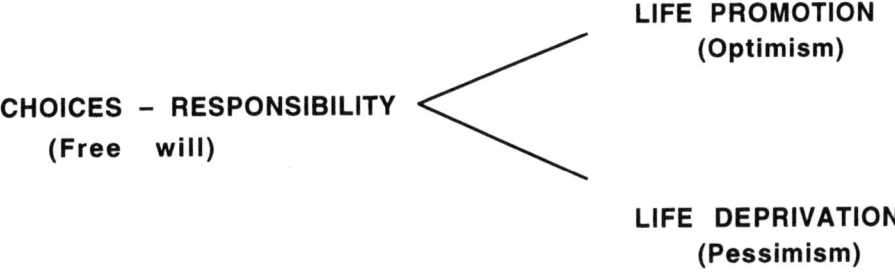

Figure 1: Everyone is his own responsibility – choose what you want to be.

Activation of our healing potential gives rise to a *healing response* (figure 2). The healing response can be initiated either primarily by inner forces in us (will, wish, hope – conscious or unconscious, listening to ourselves through meditation, relaxation etc.). Or secondarily by outer circumstances, for example represented by a lucky meeting with the right doctor, alternative therapist or other person, or events in our life such as falling in love, getting the right job, winning the lottery etc. Such outer circumstances might give rise to a sufficient stimulation of the indispensable inner forces which might not be strong enough in the first place to initiate a healing response. Lack or deprivation of the preconditions for manifestation of the healing potential means a decay of life processes resulting in sickness – and eventually death!

---

3   Which might be said among others to consist of a stress potential (fight and flight), an altruistic potential (love, empathy), a reproduction potential (sexuality), an artistic potential, a spiritual potential, etc.

Level 1
OUTER STIMULATING FACTORS OR INSPIRING CIRCUMSTANCES
(Therapeutic actions (specific or non-specific) in connection with orthodox or alternative therapy, inspiration from other persons, books and different branches of art, falling in love, have something to live for and being needed, high job satisfaction etc.)

Level 2
INNER STIMULATING FACTORS
(Wish to live, will to survive, optimism, positive feeling for life, spiritual and religious experiences and beliefs, moral and ethical motivation, personal insight in own inner nature through meditation and relaxation etc.)

Level 3
THE HEALING RESPONSE
(Strengthening of immune system, activation of balancing forces in physiology, stopping doing injurious things to one-self and others etc.)

Figure 2: The healing response may start at level 1 or 2, but is often mingled. In all circumstances the healing response has to be started from within the person by inner stimulating factors to become manifest.

The Essentials: Empathy, Tender Love and Care

If all healing, when it comes right down to it, is in fact *self-healing* and health is based on *self-regulation* (homeostasis, balance), in other words comes from within the individual – what is then the difference between orthodox medicine and alternative medicine in supporting the self-healing of nature?

If we instead of looking at what *divides* the two areas looked at what *unites* them, I find that an essential common ground ought to be our mutual interest in helping people by stimulating their inner strength or healing power.

My proposal is that we, in diagnosis and therapy, first and foremost consider the individual characteristics of each fellow being/patient and state that the treatment works through stimulation of the self-healing capacity of the organism. The investigation of this statement may well present an intriguing challenge for the development of future medicine.

Maybe we do not need to investigate so much after all, as it is a common experience that the best way of stimulating the inner healing powers of our fellow human beings is through tender love and care: the old virtues of empathy and caring. As doctors and therapists of all kinds we are here to serve rather than to ask : "What is in it for me?" We ought to forget a little about money, status and fame and fighting about whether we are "official" or "alternative" in our search for helping others.

The word *panacea,* a nonexistent outer remedy for illness, comes from the name of the old Greek medical god Aesculapius' daughter. The placebo response, understood as a self-healing response, might be the real panacea which mankind has searched for so long outside of himself.

It is said: "Doctor heal thyself." But everybody – not only doctors – should heal themselves! We should all be our own best healer! Self-healing patients make the doctor superfluous. Those patients who are not, often make the doctor seem to be *Dr. Helpless!*

List of contributors

David Aldridge, Professor
Medizinische Fakultät,
Universität Witten/Herdecke
Alfred Herrhausen Str. 50
58448 Witten, Germany
e-mail: davida@uni-wh.de

Toke Barfod, medical student
Institut for Almen Medicin,
Aarhus University
Høegh-Guldbergsgade 8, 2.,
8000 Århus C, Denmark
e-mail: TB@alm.aau.dk

Madeleine Bastide,
Professor Immunology
Laboratoire d'Immunologie et Parasitologie, Université Montpellier I
Faculté de Pharmacie,
15, avenue Charles Flahault
34060 Montpellier Cedex 1, France

Espen Braathen,
Cand.mag., M.Phil, M.Sc., M. Sc.
Central Nowegian Competence Centre
for Substance Abuse,
Breivikveien 54-56
6018 Aalesund, Norway

Vigdis Moe Christie, socionom
Department Group for Community
Medicine,
Section for Medical Anthropology,
University of Oslo
Postboks 1130 Blindern
0317 Oslo, Norway

Bent Eikard, MD, anesthesiology
Klostervej 8, Vemmetofte
4640 Fakse, Denmark
e-mail: beikard@pip.dknet.dk

Motzi Eklöf
Institute of Tema Research,
Department of Health and Society,
Linköping University
581 83 Linköping, Sweden

Elisabeth Hsu, Dr.
Faculty of Oriental Studies,
University of Cambridge
Sidgwick Ave.
Cambridge CB3 9DA, United Kingdom

Helle Johannessen, Associate Professor
Almagervej 2,
4291 Ruds Vedby, Denmark

Robert Lafaille, Ph.D
International Institute for Advanced
Health Studies
Kardinaal Mercierlei, 26,
2600 Antwerp, Belgium

Agnès Lagache, Professor Philosophy
PhD (letters), "Prix de Rome" literature
5, Rue Ste Anastase
75003 Paris, France

Dieter Melchart, Dr. med.
Projekt 'Münchener Modell',
Ludwig-Maximilians-Universität
Kaiserstraße 9
80801 München, Germany

Aase Krogh Mortensen, stud. anthro.
Department of Ethnography and Social Anthropology, Aarhus University
Moesgård, 8270 Højbjerg, Denmark

Phillip A. Nicholls, Dr.
Division of Sociology,
Staffordshire University
College Road
Stoke-on-Trent, Staffordshire ST4 2DE, United Kingdom

Rebecca Rees,
Audit and outcomes coordinator
Research Council for Complementary Medicine (RCCM)
60 Great Ormond Street
London WC1N 3JF, United Kingdom
e-mail: rccm@gn.apc.org

Vilhelm Schjelderup,
General Practitioner
Sjøboden 1, 3110 Tønsberg, Norway

Ursula Sharma, Dr.
Professor in Sociology
School of Education and Social Sciences, University of Derby
Derby DE3 5GX, United Kingdom

Mary Ryan-Thorup, phd candidate
Institute of Anthropology,
University of Copenhagen
Frederiksholms Kanal 4
1220 Copenhagen K, Denmark
e-mail: mary.ryan.thorup@anthro.ku.dk

Tobias Waltjen
Wissensarchiv - Study Group on Documentation and Research in Integrated Medicine, c/o Wiener Internationale Akademie für Ganzheitsmedizin
Kurbadstr. 8,
A-1108 Wien, Austria
e-mail: twaltjen@ping.at